The Tai Chi Cane

太极拳手杖

Author – Sifu Bob

Copyright

Text and Pictures Copyright © 2019 Robert G. Downey

All Rights Reserved

Public domain Photos from Gray's Anatomy

(If you do not have a volume get one!)

Dedication

To all my many teachers

Grandmaster William C. C. Chen

Grandmaster Liang Tse Tung

Master Chan Bun-Piac 川

Dr. John P. Painter

Thomas Morgan for asking all the questions and challenging the answers.

And the many more

Remember as T.T. always said, "you need teachers, and you need books"

Grandmaster Chen says "Trust Yourself"

Preface

The cane is not an original Tai Chi Chuan weapon. The original weapons of Tai Chi Chuan are or were – the knife, the sword, the staff, and the spear and taught in that order. As Tai Chi Chuan grew, many weapons were adapted to the methods and theories of Tai Chi Chuan. Grandmaster Liang was a traditionalist in his Tai Chi Chuan but studied many things that interested him and many he incorporated into his teachings.

Grandmaster Liang had a friend and fellow student of the arts at the school and adapted from him a Shaolin Cane form and a version of the five Animals Chi Gong. The cane fits into Tai Chi Chuan with little modification. The only thing he did not do is put a scarf on one end of it and challenge us to make it fly.

Since the Cane was part of Grandmaster Liang teachings, the volumes published by Golden Flower Internal Arts added this topic. .

There are been modifications over the years but it is close to true to his teachings. The essence of Tai Chi Chuan with the workings of the footwork and the body movements are in this form.

Teaching a set in a book is very difficult but books last long and are easy to go review. Therefore, we hope that this will be of value in the reader's progress in the internal arts. This is a basic book to provide the basics of using a cane or similar weapon. If time permits, publishing a second volume on the more refined aspects is scheduled. In the meantime, look for the other Internal Arts Series volumes on Amazon.

Table of Contents

Tai Chi Cane

The Cane was never one of the original Tai Chi weapons. It was as many other weapons assimilated into the Internal Arts. Grandmaster Liang added it to the Tai Chi Dance School in the '80s from a Shaolin Cane set. He liked weapons. Grandmaster Liang walked all over town with a cane. His cane went click, click, and click as he put weight on it. Only those in the know knew that it was a sword cane. The noise came from the looseness of the blade in its sheath as the cane reset with his weight.

Grandmaster Liang taught that the cane had not only the brutal impact of the Knife but the delicate movement of the sword and that to use a cane it needed to be soft and slow until the energy permeated the cane. So when practicing with the cane, use the ideas and principles of Tai Chi Chuan to make it soft and energetic.

If using a cane for practical use – a walking cane – prevent slipping by using a tip on the end of the cane. This can be just to flatten the end or install a felt or rubber end. A copper pipefitting can be fitted to protect the edges.

Canes, Canes and more Canes

Canes can take on very elaborate designs or can simply be a piece of branch strong enough to support the body. Looking at the designs available now as well as those used in various times of history can be a fascinating journey. Find a cane that makes sense. Have many canes for the many practice sessions needed.

A cane is any material that fits in the hand and reaches from the hand when it is at the waist and stops at or near the ground at the side of the foot. Canes will vary depending on the size of the player and their hand size. A cane material can be of any manner of materials but must be strong enough to take and give the force of a blow. Remember that the cane form is training for picking up anything of similar size for defense.

The cane is a simple piece of wood or something made with care and decorated with carvings and unique handles. Remember that a cane should allow the hands to slide up and down its length so decorations should be ingrain not outside obstructing the movement of the hands. Wood is one of the most common materials for a cane. Hardwood is preferred to prevent breaking. One extremely strong material that is readily available is ash. An old garden tool handle or a purchased replacement can become a cane. A simple sanding and an oil rub make a beautiful useful weapon. Taking it for a walk, it helps to provide familiarity with it but provides instant protection.

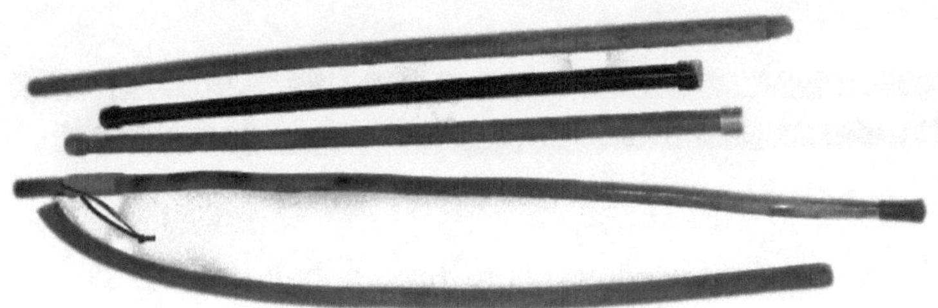

Making a cane

The handle of a gardening tool can easily make a cane. A simple handsaw will cut the handle off. Cut as close to the tool end as possible. The end of the handle rounded makes a good handle. Now put that handle on the ground and grip the cane with the hand at the side of the leg. The top end of the hand should be marked on the canes as the appropriate length – put the rounded end on the ground. Using the saw cut off the rest of the material making sure that the cut is square. A file and some sandpaper rounds the cut edge. Lightly sand the rest of the cane and apply a wood oil to preserve the wood. This creates the first and maybe the best working cane. Designs carved on the cane provide for artist flair. Canes do not have to be smooth. A knot protruding can add to the impact and aid in catching another weapon. Just be sure that the knot does not weaken the cane too much.

A second project is to get a piece of heavy walled 1 ½ "PVC pipe which can be purchased in 4' lengths at a building supply store. Get end caps for each end. Cut to length as previously detailed. Some batting tape, available at any sporting goods store, added one end creates a grip. Adjust the cane's weight with the addition of material inside to adjust the weight. Sand added to the cane can provide heft. A can of foam insulation can aid in maintaining the location of the sand in the cane. Remember that this cane is a good two-person practice tool and weight may not be a good idea since it can add to the impact. This cane does make a quick cane that is inexpensive and having a number around will aid in practice.

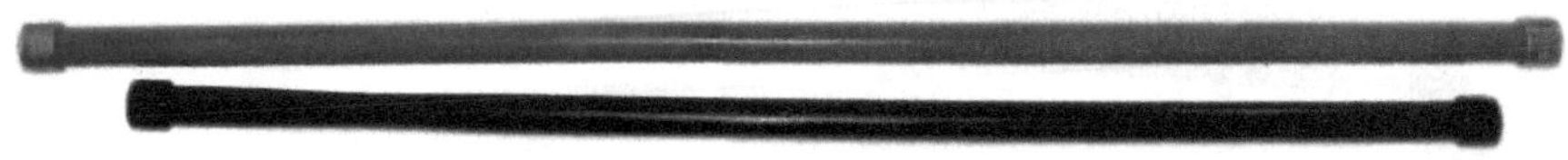

These are two simple methods to have a cane to start practicing. A favorite is always close at hand.[1]

Attacking methods

Strikes

This is an internal use of the cane as a weapon. There are differences between the Internal and External Arts. The external use of a cane uses the force of the swing to create the impact strength of the strike. The force is generated by increasing the speed of the cane towards the impact location. This requires a large and quick swing.

The Internal use of the cane also uses speed but the impact is a matter of intent and focus. An Internal swing can be face but will only touch the body with light force unless the player defines a strike. Soft and loose is the mantra of the internal arts. In this manner, a swing intercepted will result in a soft impact. This impact can then develop into another attack. Only when the strike is defined is the body connected. Then the energy of the speed of the strike PLUS the internal energy generated by the focused energy through the root and the body determines the impact of the cane. This is not an easy action to develop. It is what is needed to train in the use of an internal art. This is the softness and Tai Chi Chuan. Practice by attacking the target and only touching it lightly. Do it slowly at first and then develop speed. Focused energy, Fa Jin, is practiced later. A full discussion of Fa Jin in the Internal Arts is available in the Golden Arts Series.

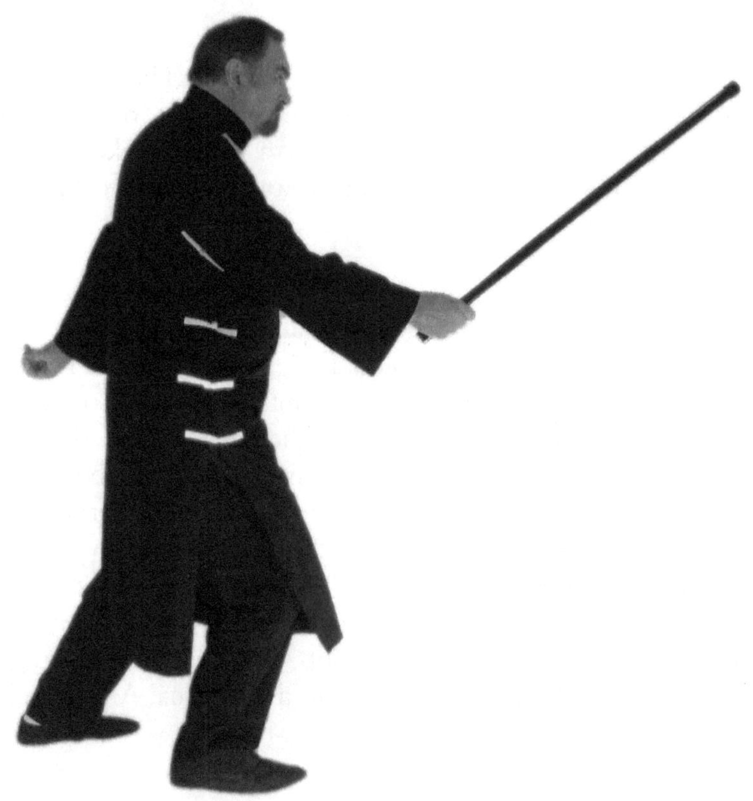

Underhand

Horizontal

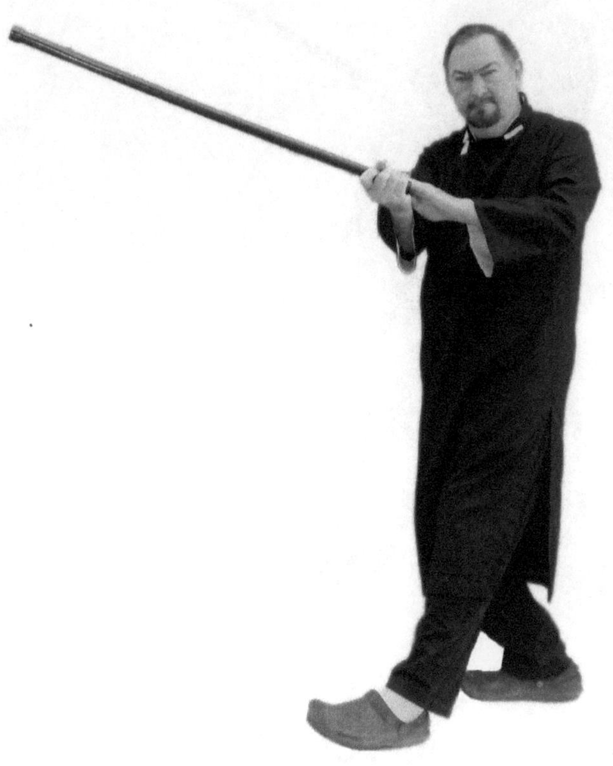

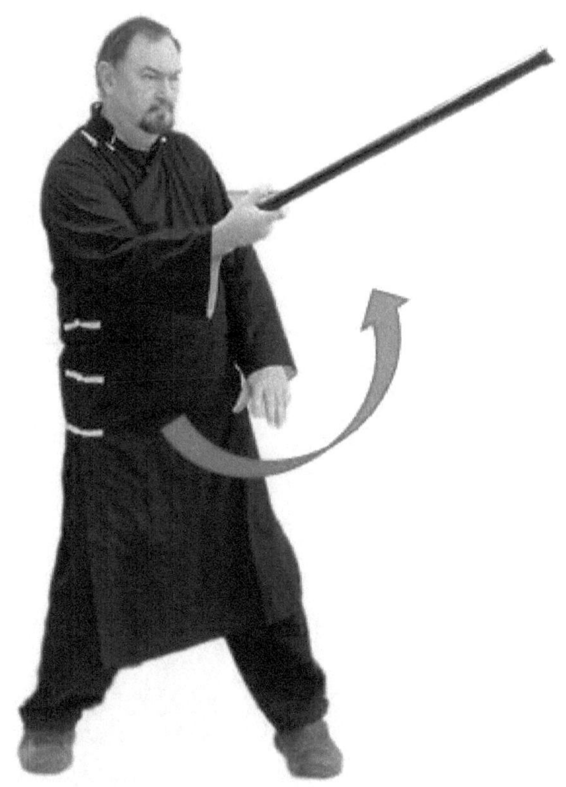

Diagonal Upper Strike

Poke or Stab

A poke and a stab are just about the same thing. About the only difference is the intent. A poke is more an action to create another action from the opponent. A stab has enough force to end the encounter, many times supported by the secondary hand.

An attack with the cane end when being held in the hand by the end creates a weapon that can attack using the opposite end of the cane. When done with the primary hand alone the attack is usually called a poke and although it can have a detrimental effect on the opponent creates another opening such as lowering the guard to protect against the poke and the player then attacks with an overhand strike into the exposed area.

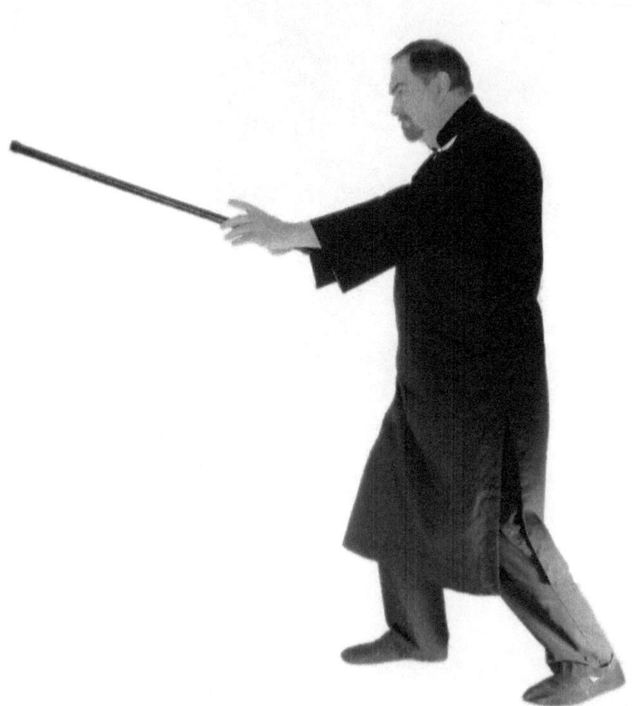

A supported attack with the end of the cane has the palm of the support hand on the top of the cane or at least grabbing over the gripping hand to provide more force in the attack. The Supported Attack aims at vulnerable spots on the opponent such as internal organs or joints.

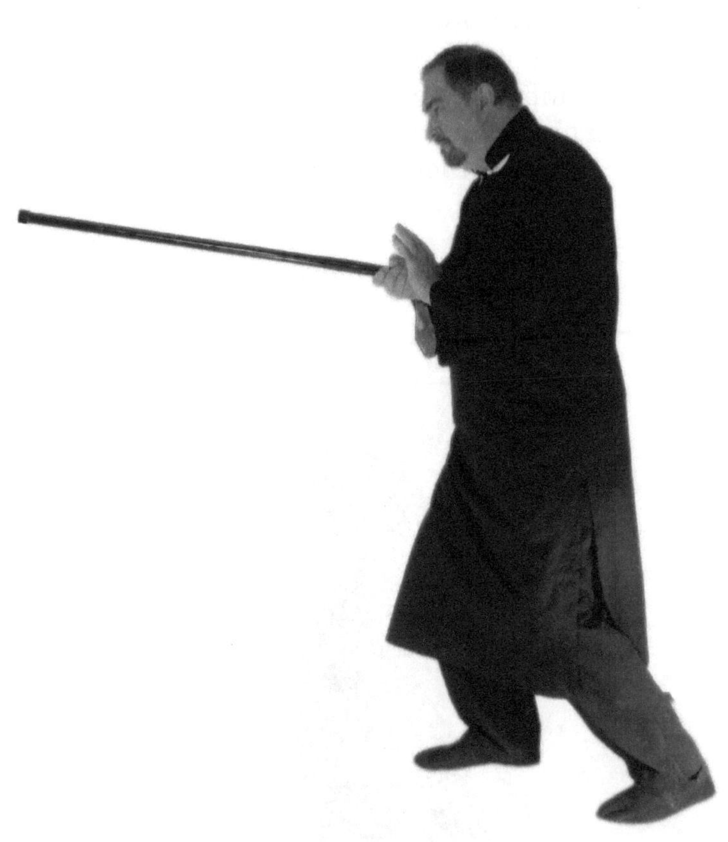

Two-Handed Strike

Standing Cane

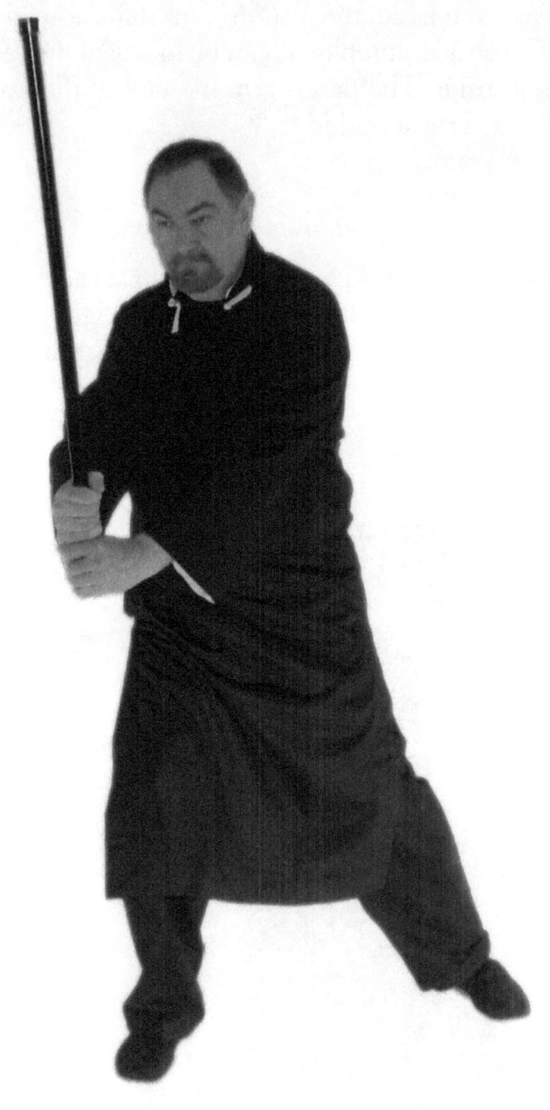

The first two-handed strike makes the cane take on the power of a bat. A single hand does not have enough gripping power for a standing posture so the second hand helps to hold a standing cane. The player can then use as much force as they can generate to attack the opponent. Since there is a large amount of force, the actual attacking location can be less specific and the cane just used for clubbing actions. This does not mean that specific targets are not used but if that target is missed the action can still cause the opponent substantial damage. The strikes and blocks can be in any of the four directions as in the single-handed strike. The hands grip the end of the cane as if a bat but the opposite end in a vertical position.

Double Hand

The second two-handed strike is with one hand at each end of the cane. The middle of the cane becomes the weapon's attacking edge. Note in this picture that the weight shifts to the front foot and the heel raises to get more power into the strike.

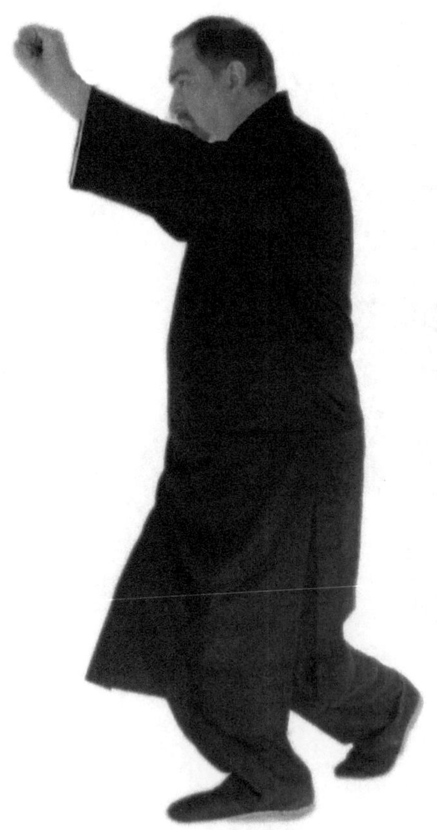

Defensive Methods

Single Handed Block

Holding the cane in one hand is a standard movement in the use of the cane. The action of swinging the cane and attacking the opponent causes a large amount of force to be in that movement of the cane. The player can attempt to meet this energy force on force but the stronger force overcomes the weaker and requires the player to exert a large amount of energy. Using the cane in one hand and meeting the force of the opponent at an angle will allow a far less exertion of force and will direct the attack away from the player. This is the standard for use of the cane in preventing an attack with the one-handed grip. Many movements will use the empty hand on the full hand's wrist to provide support.

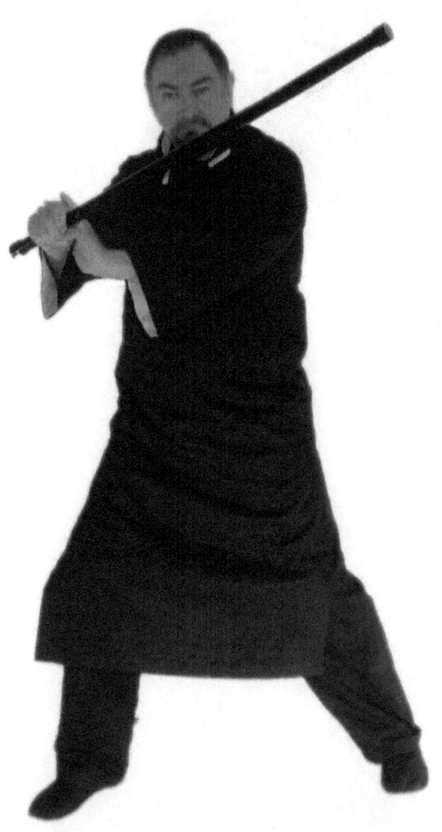

Two-Handed Block

The two-handed block uses the two handed strike but reversed. The cane meets the energy and redirect and absorbs it rather than meeting force with force.

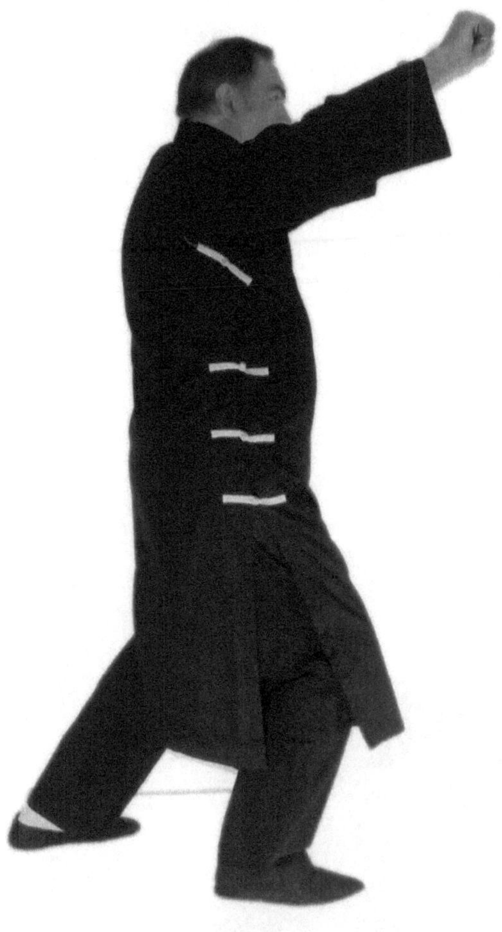

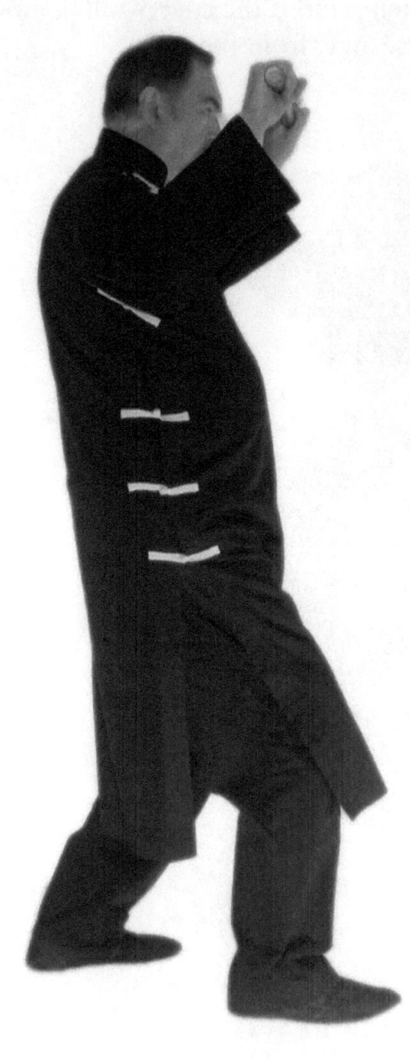

Two Handed Deflection

The second two-handed block with each hand holding an end of the cane again meets force with direction. This block does not overpower the attack but halts the direction and then redirect the energy with a movement in the hands turning the attacker's force away from the body.

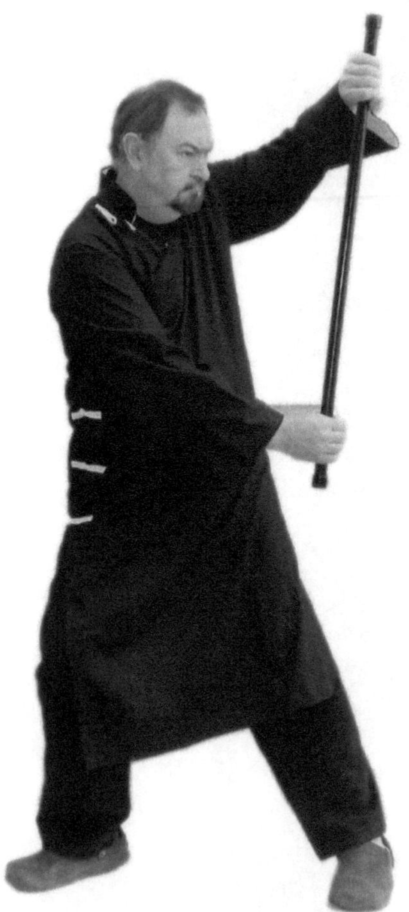

The weak hand (empty)

One hand in any use of a single weapon will be empty of a weapon but is still a weapon whether defensive or offensive when used properly. The weak hand in the cane form is for striking, grasping the opponent, supporting the attacking wrist, or grasping the cane to become part of the battle. Never ignore the weak hand! Always use it as an integral part of the set. The practice sets discuss many applications. Note in the many pictures that the empty hand is always active.

Practice Sets

There are a number of easily learned practice sets. We will start with the single player practice movements then move to two-person practice movements and then two-person practice sets. These are just the basics and with training and practice, many more and longer sets are developed. All references will be to player A and Player B to distinguish who is moving. All movements start with the basic stance and the cane in a ready position.

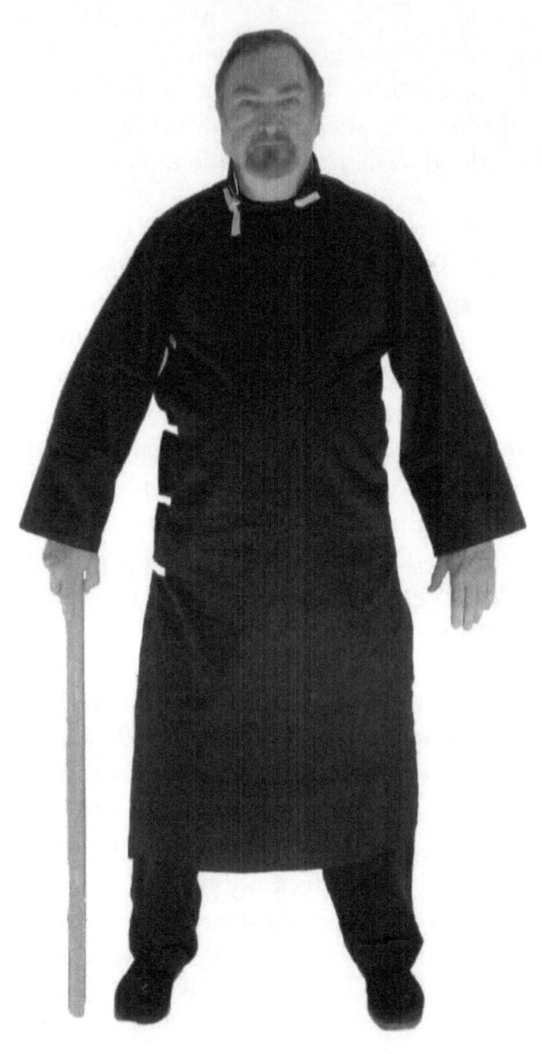

Posts and targets

Even though the cane can be an aggressive weapon not needing accuracy, the practice on targets is an important part to get full use of the weapon and direct the energy properly to the target. Trees are frequently targets but hitting repeatedly will cause damage. Use a 4" post either square or round and set it into the ground. Use paint to create targets for focus. A round post is gentler on a cane. A square post can serve the dual purpose of weapon and hand work.

A hanging bag, either commercially made or homemade, is an effective target. If the bag is hanging with no attachment to the floor, it will move with strikes and provide emphasis on seeking the target at the opinion time. Bags can have tape or paint added to them to provide targets as in a static post.

Energy use in hitting with a cane can take on two principles of Tai Chi Chuan – an Jin or fa Jin. To describe these would take volumes but a quick discussion is important to keep the cane an internal weapon. An Jin is the application of force over an extended period. This uses the whole body as in all Tai Chi practices but starts with the impact on the target and extends into the duration of the strike. Fa Jin is to apply the whole body energy over a very short period. The effect of each of these impacts is different but each has its purpose in the use of a weapon. As an example, the standing cane is more likely to use An Jin to move the opponent's weapon away from the player. Fa Jin can be used in a single-handed strike since apply the energy is in one moment and not needed to extend where the wrist can give out on extended high power attack over time.

Now, it is important to get back to where the softness of internal arts comes in with the use of the cane. Using the one-handed strike as an example, the action moves the cane from one position to the target and then the strike. The motion to the target must be soft though directed to the target with accuracy. If the opponent intercepts the cane during the action, the two canes should not meet with force. The attack should simply use the opponent's energy to redirect the action and then add that energy to an attack at another target on the opponent. This is the softness of Tai Chi Chuan where all movements are soft until, as to paraphrase the Professor, applied with the appropriate level of force.

Understand and practice these paragraphs in all phases of Tai Chi Arts. Using these techniques, the practice of the cane will help develop the internal energy to make the mind and body healthy. The volume on training tools and techniques will go into detail on these issues.

Single Player Sets

Single player sets imagine a player of similar stature standing in front to allow for proper movements and points of impact.

Circles

CIRCLES

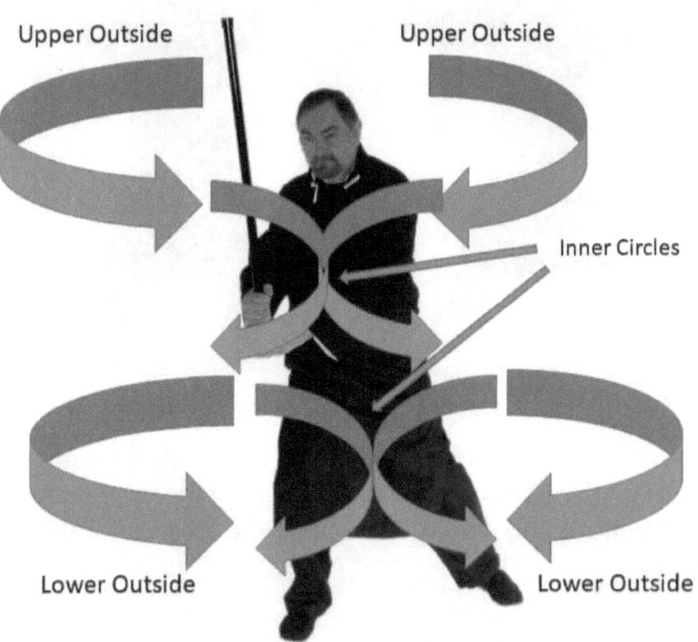

Circles are in relation to the forward foot, the strong arm, and the centerline. In the example below, the right leg and right arm are extended. The outside starts at the beginning of the circle. The outside circles are starting with the energy coming out of the center line moving away from the body for an outside circle and the inside circle has the energy going into the center line at the beginning and then moving away. It is not overly important at the beginning – just learn the circles. Advanced training actually uses these ideas to aid in the circulation of the energy – the advanced volume.

Outward high circle

The player starting from the ready position swings the cane out and in a circular motion up to the head height of the opponent. The cane should be under control and stop movement at the location of the imaginary opponent's head.

Inward high circle

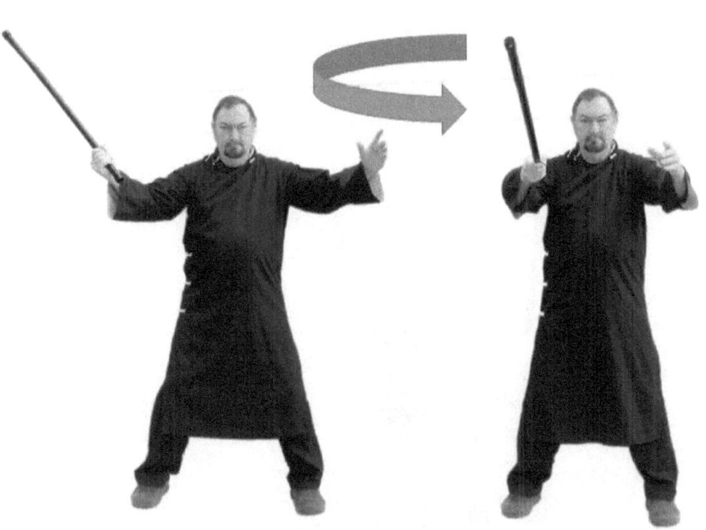

Upper Outer Circle Strike

The player starting from the ready position swings the cane across the body and up in a circular motion to the head height of the opponent. The cane should be under control and stop movement at the location of the imaginary opponent's head.

Outward lower circle

The player swings the cane out and down from its ready position and stops at the opponent's knee. In this and the next movement, the attacked

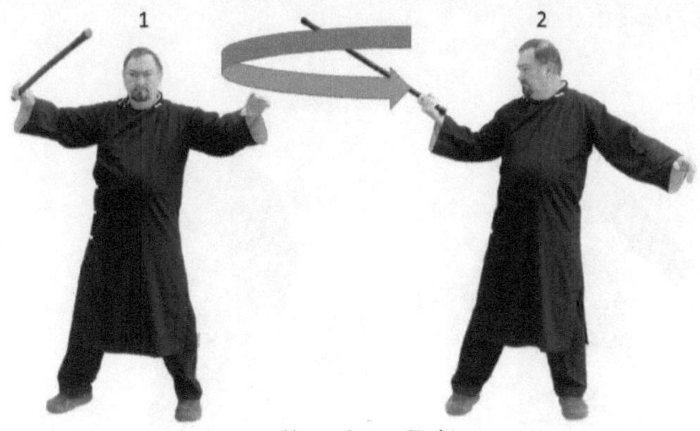

Upper Inner Circle

position could be whichever knee is in a forward position or the outside if in a horse stance.

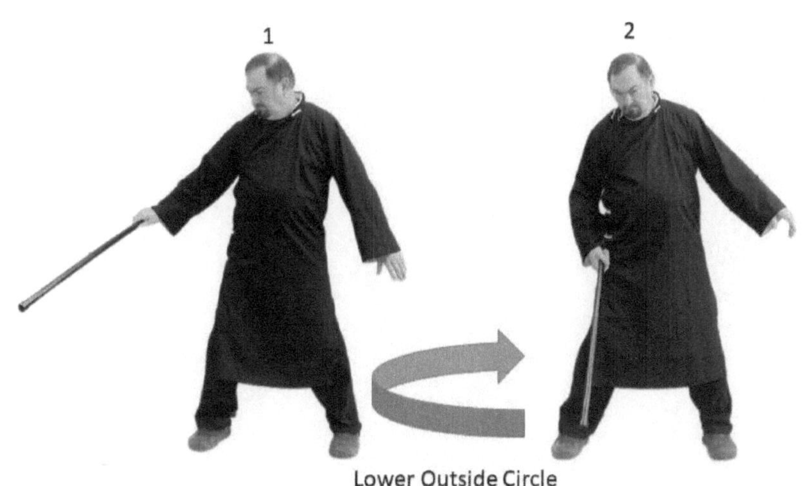

Lower Outside Circle

Inward lower circle

The player swings the cane across the body and down from its ready position and stops at the opponent's knee. This attack takes on two movements. The attack can be on the first part of the circle – the inward movement or on the completion of the circle. The second attack can use either a forehand or a backhand attack. Practice all.

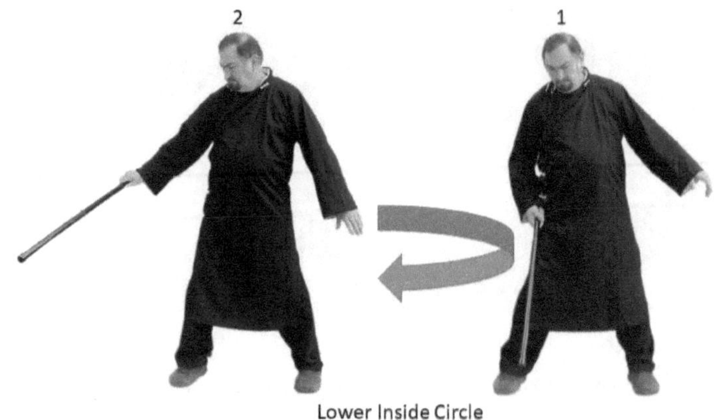

Lower Inside Circle

The player swings the cane down and back then up and over to attack the top of the head or the shoulder of the opponent. The circle can be on either side of the body. The actions are soft but fast with the cane held loosely until impact.

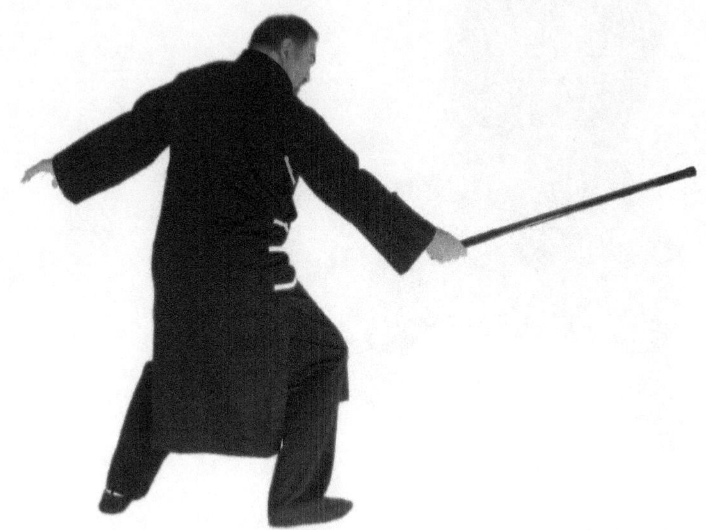

Underhand Attack

The player swings the cane down and to the front and then up to attack the opponent with the attacking point being any exposed part of the body including the knee, hip, ribs or under the arm.

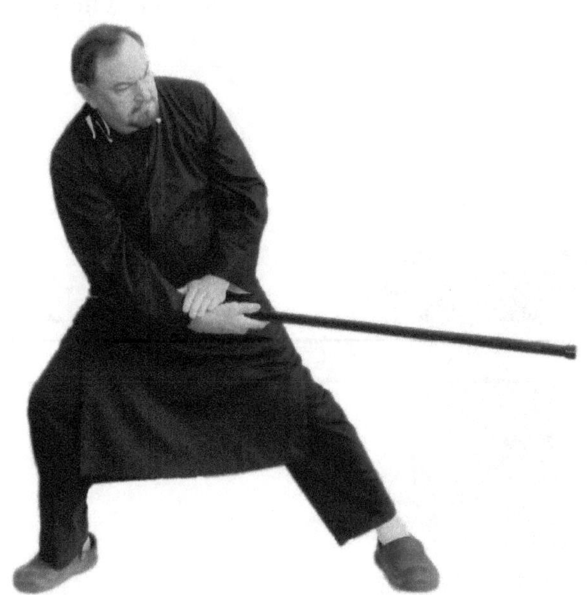

Standing Cane Attack

Inside

The player raises the cane up to a standing position in front of the body. The weak hand comes in to add to the support of the cane. The player turns the waist[2] to the left bringing the cane across the body .and shifts the weight to the rear leg. Standing cane attacks the arms of the opponent.

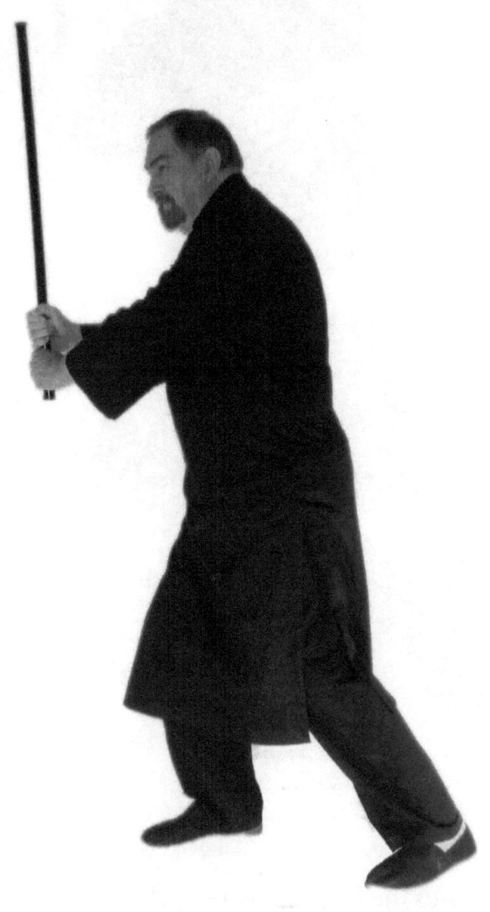

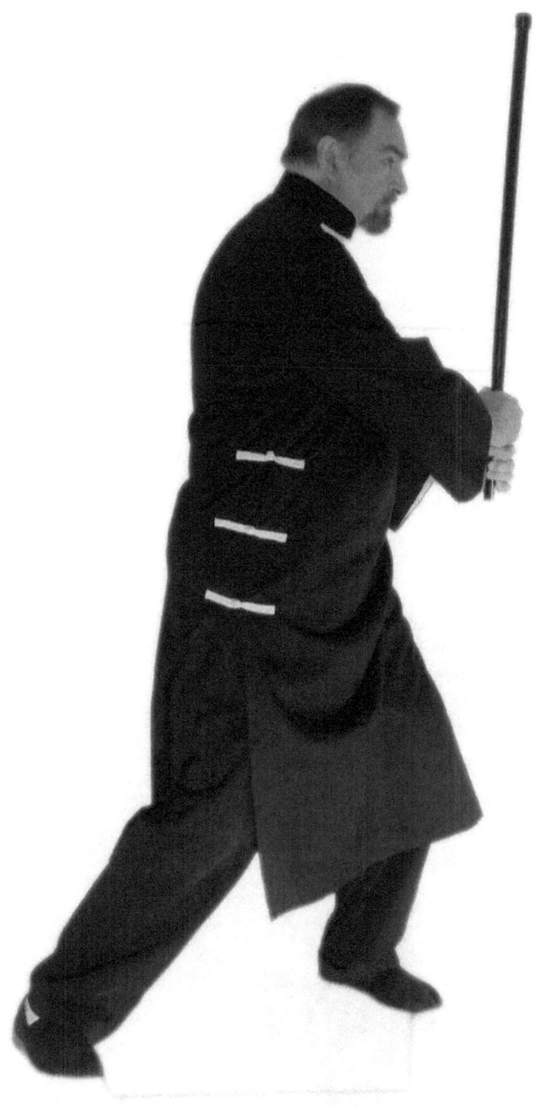

The player raises the cane up to a standing position in front of the body. The weak hand comes in to add to the support of the cane. The player turns the waist to the right bringing the cane across the body.

Two-handed Attack

The player brings the cane up with the end moving across the body as the weak hand reaches up and grabs the end of the cane. The cane moves to a horizontal position at a level of the eyebrows allowing the player to see under the cane but protecting the player's head. The player then strikes out at the opponent using the center of the cane to strike.

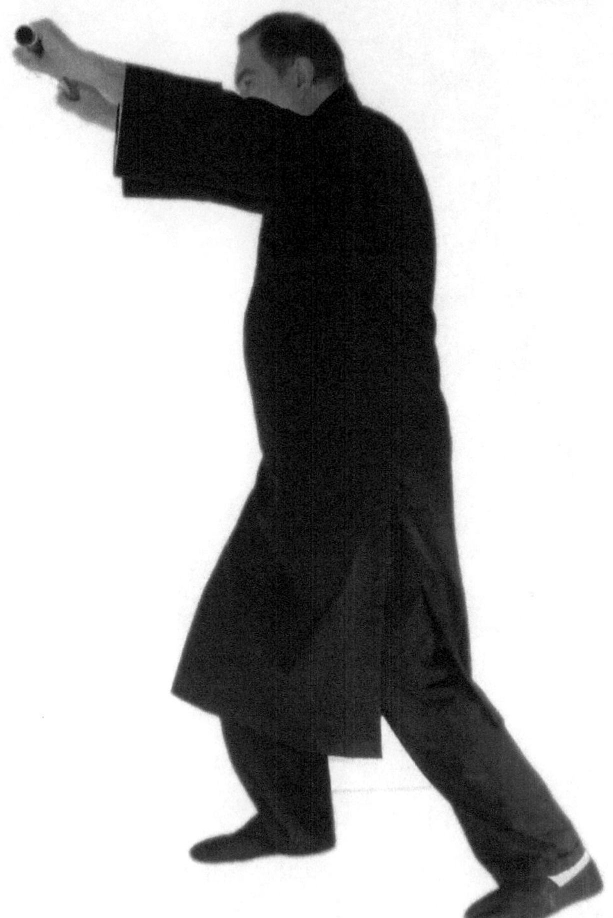

All the previous practices are from a static stance. Stepping, described below, allows for the development of movement in each exercise.

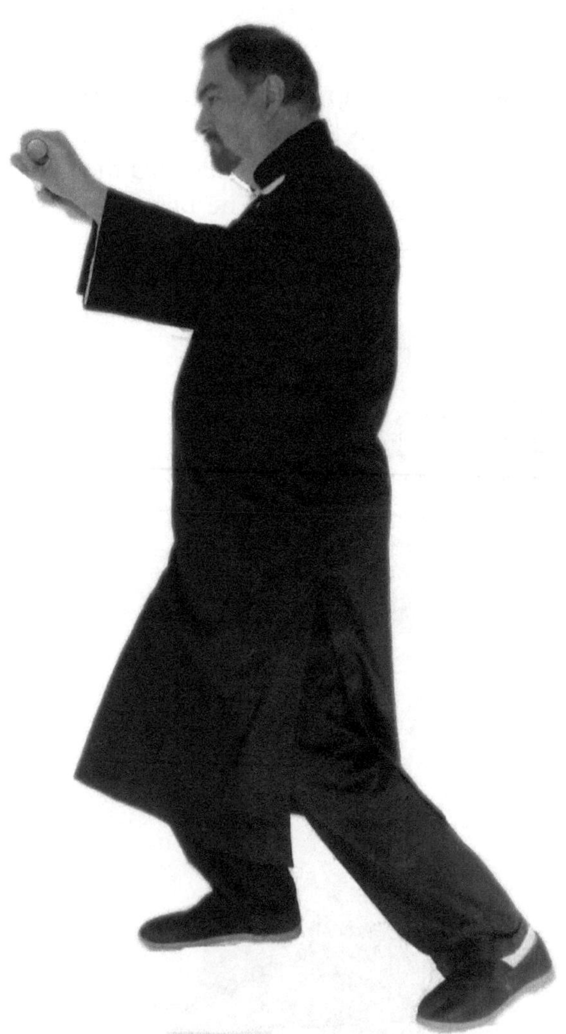

Stepping and Stances

Horse stance

A horse stance, named after riding the horse position, has both feet pointing forward and the feet just inside of shoulder width. The weight is divided unevenly. This prevents the curse of double weighting and allows for the rapid shift of weight and movement of the body. Usually, the weight is favored 70% to 30%. A better way of gauging the weight distribution is to remove weight on the unweighted foot until it can be picked up. The weighted foot usually holds the weapon in a ready stance.

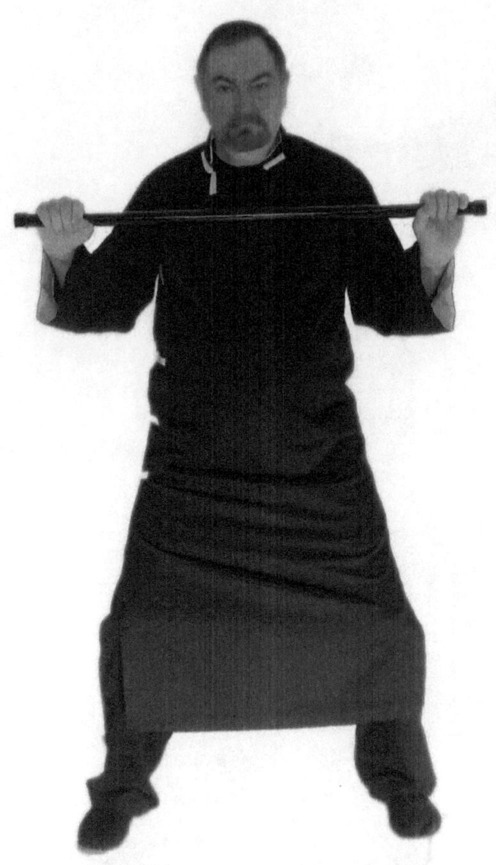

The footsteps forward and is planted and the weight shifts forward into the foot. Transfer the weight before any action. Either foot can step forward. The thigh of the rear leg should be vertical.

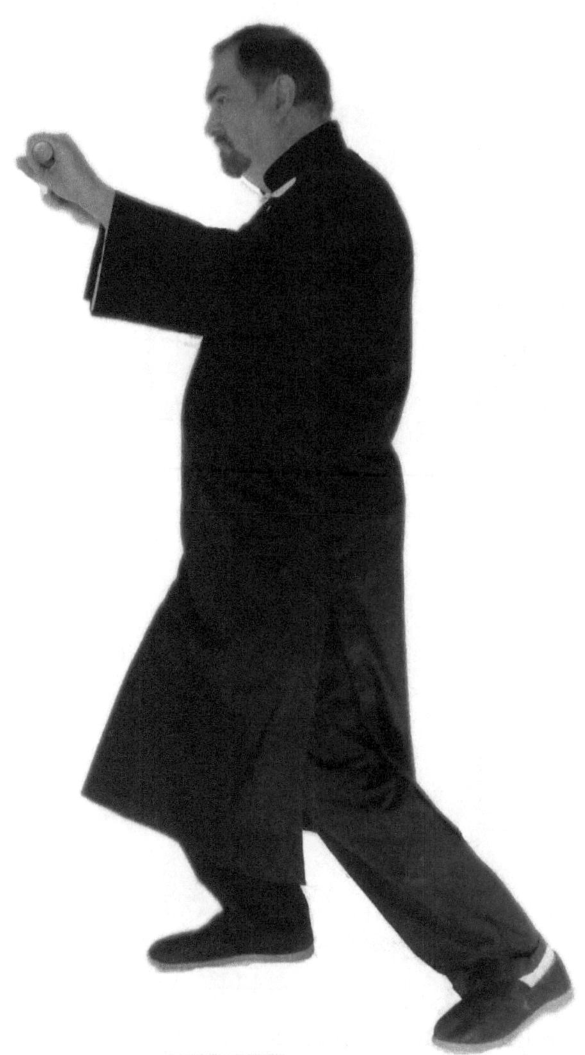

Bow Stance Back Weighted

The foot steps forward to a normal stepping position but the weight does not shift into that foot. When the blow is struck, the unweighted foot gives the player the opportunity to move immediately after the blow.

Cat Stance

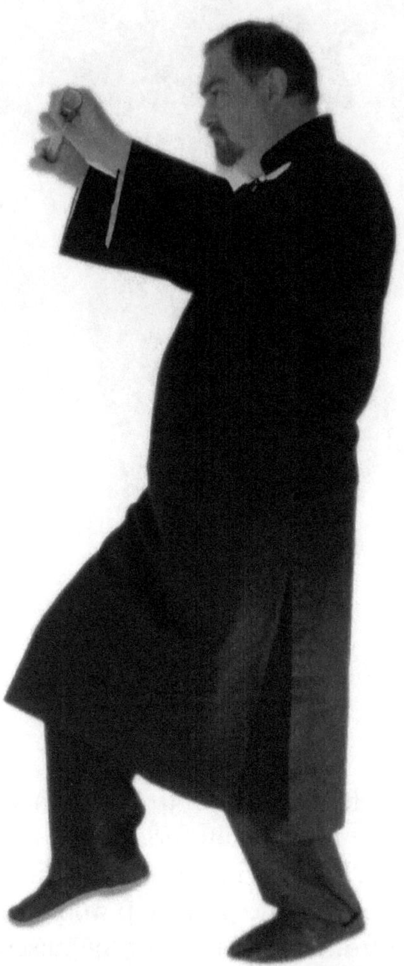

The step is to the toe touches the ground and the heel remains elevated. This can be a testing stance for footing but also provides a ready position for a kick following the attack.

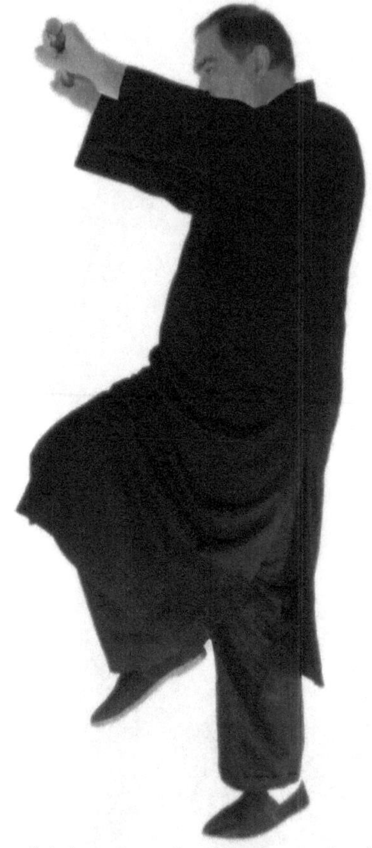

In this position, the thigh raises the leg from the knee and the foot held up. This can be a movement in preparation for a follow-up kick or can be to avoid a strike to the leg or knee. If practicing the later, it is important to practice with a prior step as well as without. The prior step would be small and quick to allow some distance away from the position of the raised leg. The lack of the first step should include the nesting of the foot into the opposite knee to aid in the prevention of injury to the weighted knee.

Backward Step

The unweighted leg steps backward and the weight shifts to the back foot and the now unweighted leg comes back in either a raised step or one more backward step.

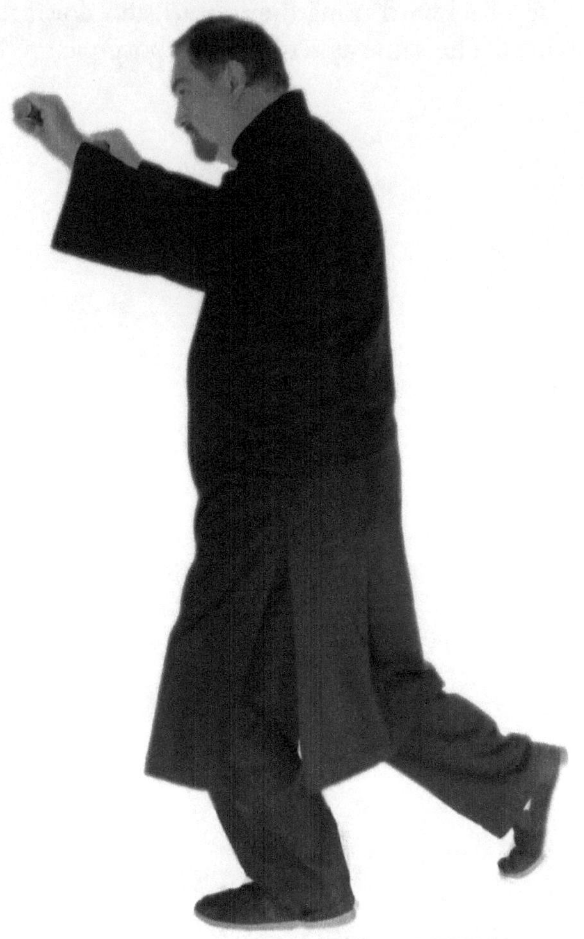

Turning steps

A simple turn involves the action of turning the foot out or in compared to the centerline of the current position. A smaller step allows the player to maintain balance during the stepping. The foot turns out or in at an angle of 30 – 90 degrees as the foot steps down and the weight shifts into the foot. The player can also step backward using the foot to step down toe first and then shifting into the heel. The same as seen in the above picture but with the foot at an angle.

There are two methods of turning around – the weighted turn and the multistep turn. The weighted turn – spinning on a weighted foot is elegant but not often practical. Footwear and footing must be adequate to allow for the spinning. Many times one or the other will grab preventing the complete turn. This can provide the attacker an opportunity to attack the player in a vulnerable position.

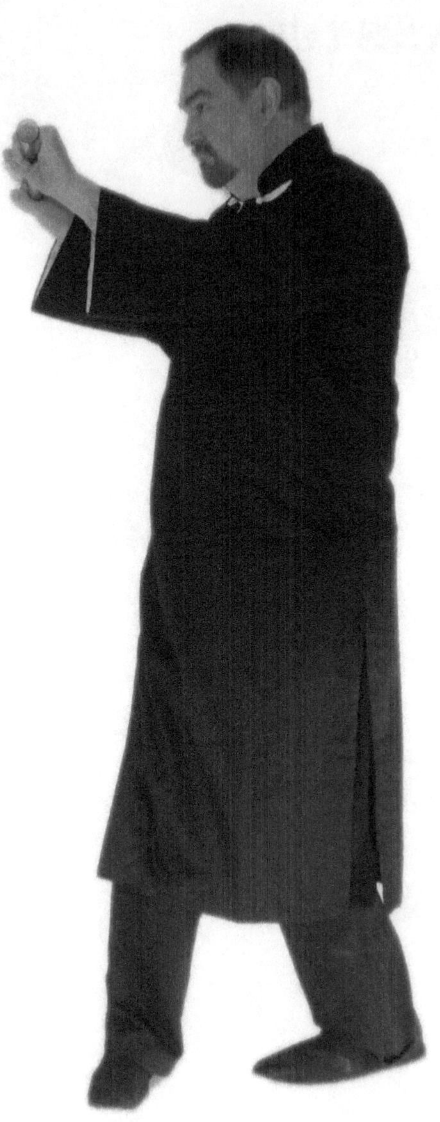

The multistep turn – often called the old man's turn – provides more secure footing and attacks and defends at 360 degrees around the body. This uses the four-step movement and at any of those steps, attacks and defensive actions present options. These movements are completely broken down in the Tai Chi volumes[3] but practice and see how to use them in any footing situation.

OLD MAN'S TURN

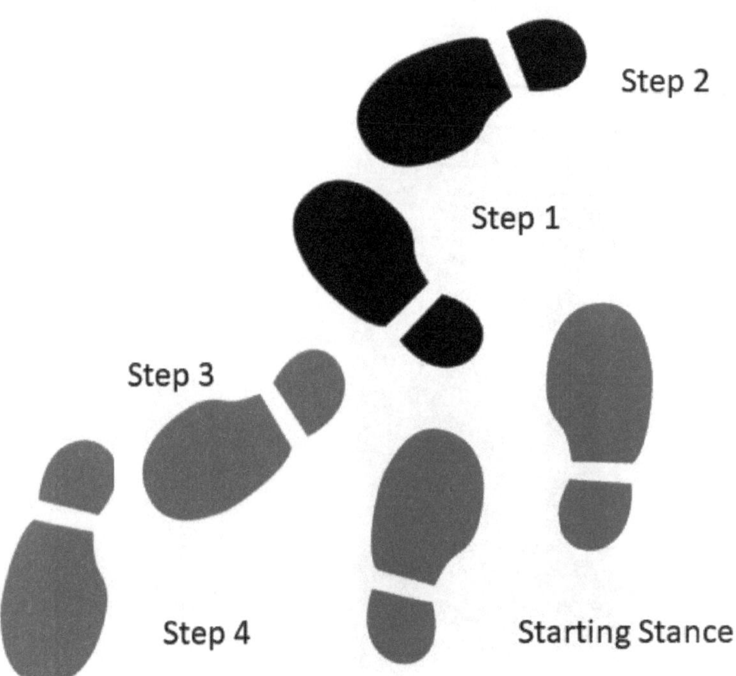

Cross Step

A cross step is a common step in martial arts allowing for a lowering of the posture while maintaining a strong posture. The stepping foot can either cross the front or to the rear of the static foot. The step creates an X in the legs. The weight shifts with the step into the stepping leg or settled into the static leg. The upper body must stay erect over the weighted leg as the weight is shifted and the knees bent as the body is lowered. The knee must stay over the foot to prevent damage to the ligaments of the knee.

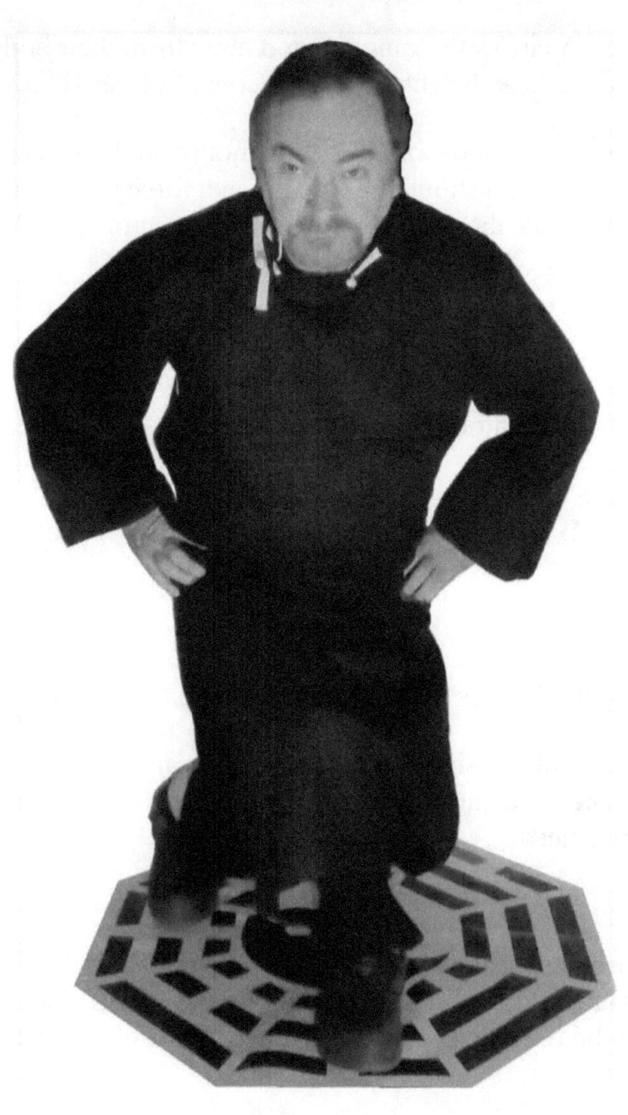

Two-person practice

Two-person practice must be done with care and consider the use of safety equipment[4]. Practice movements in slow motion. This is an internal cane so the importance is to develop the energy from the body to play the cane and not external force. Both players should start in the ready position. Each player should measure their location in reference to the other player and all practice strikes should be well in front of each player to prevent accidental strikes and resulting injury.

Outward high circle

Player A circles the cane out and away from their body and then back into a position at head height directly in front of player B.

Player B responds with the same motion and connects with Player A's cane. The connection should be with enough force to feel the connection but not enough to shake the opponent's teeth! This is practice. When after a good period the energy of the strike can be increased.

Inward high circle

Player A circles the cane in and across their body and then back into a position at head height directly in front of player B. This is a backhand hold on the cane.

Player B responds with the same motion and connects with Player A's cane.

Outward lower circle

A circles the cane out and then down to a position at knee level of B.

B can protect using either an inward or an outward circle. The inward circle is quicker and most efficient in protecting against this strike but both should be practiced.

Inward lower circle

A circles the cane inward and down and then to the outside to strike in front of B's knee. This as in the practice exercise can be an attack on the inward circle or on the returning circle with either backhand or forehand.

B must judge when the attack is coming and protect with the attack. Each of the methods should be practiced so that requires coordination with the player to allow for the completion of the circle to practice the secondary attack and defense.

Over Hand attack

A - Swings the cane out and up and strikes down to the Level of B's head.

B can use a number of defenses. The two-hand defense with the cane held on each end and level just above the eyebrows will stop the attack. B can also bring up the cane in a diagonal movement to deflect the opponent's cane away. The two-handed standing cane can deflect the opponent's cane to the side. Practice all the movements.

Underhand Attack

A - Drops the cane down and brings it up to B's waist.

B swings the cane down and inward to intercept the upward strike and deflect it to the side. A two-handed downward strike or an outward downward strike can be used but would require added body movement. Try them and see why they are not favorable alternatives.

Standing Cane Attack

Inside

See below.

Outside

Both of these attacks hit the arms of the opponent to cause damage to their arms and/or lose their cane. To practice this set of exercises hold the cane at chest height. Defense to this attack is to move the arms out of the way. This is not a crash bang exercise unless there is movement. This movement would be to move the arms out of the way and attack the attacking cane. Techniques discussed with advanced movements in the next volume.

Two-handed Attack

A brings the cane up and across the body while bringing up the weak hand and holding the end of the cane while bringing horizontal. A pushes the cane forward to strike across the midline of **B**.

B brings up their cane in a similar manner and then allow one hand to go down and one up to a diagonal position and to intercept A's cane to prevent the strike. A single hand cane would not be strong enough to stop A's strike.

These are not all the options for practicing nor all the potential defenses. Practice and investigate each movement. Do each one slowly and with mind intent. Do not use force use energy and deflection. After learning all the movements in the horse stance, then bring in all the variations using moving steps.

Tai Chi Cane Form List

Section 1

Starting Posture	North
Swing the cane to Preparation	North
Strike Left and Kick with Right Foot	West
Strike Horizontally	North
Retreat stepping and block with two Hands	West
Step and Strike to the ears	West
Left Hook Hand, step and strike with Cane downward	West
Cover and Underhand strike	West
Step behind, sit and overhand strike with Cane	West

Section 2

Raise and Strike Left and Kick with Right Foot	East
Strike Horizontally	North
Retreat step back left foot and block with two Hands	East
Step and Strike to the ears	East
Left Hook Hand step and strike with Cane downward	East
Cover and Underhand strike	East
Step behind, sit and overhand strike with Cane	East

Section 3

Stand the cane	East
Stand and grab cane base with both hands	North

Step to the Left	Southwest
Standing cane strikes left	West
Step to the Right	North
Standing cane Strikes right	Northwest
Cover the back, Step to the Left and underhand strike	Southwest
Cover the back, Step to the Right and underhand strike	Northeast
Overhand strike left hand behind back	Northeast
Left hand goes to cane end	North
Fold cane under the Right arm	North
Spin cane to the foot	North
End of form	North

Tai Chi Cane Form Description

Grandmaster T. T. Liang developed the cane form when a Shaolin Cane was taught at the studio. Grandmaster T. T. Liang loved weapons, took the outline of the form, and made it into a Tai Chi Weapon set. It is presented here in a more defined manner to provide the player with an understanding of the practice methods. The form is divided into three sections. The first section is the left side. The left foot is the predominant front or weighted foot in the postures. The second section mirrors the first but with the right leg dominant. The third section adds some two-sided postures and wraps up the form. Enjoy.

Section 1

Starting Posture - North

The cane form beginning and ending posture is the same position. The player is standing feet pointing to the north shoulder width apart. The left hand is at waist level palm facing the south. Hold the end of the cane down to the outside of the right foot.

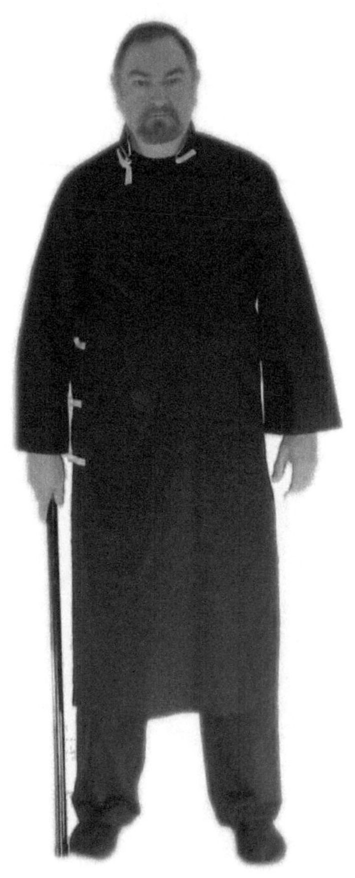

The cane is raised up with the wrist pointing North at the level of the waist and then rotated in a circle back to the same spot and then is tucked under the arm in the armpit making the cane appear somewhat hidden but in a preparatory position for use. This and the ending movement both exhibit an attack from the resting position of the cane. That is a valuable movement to remember.

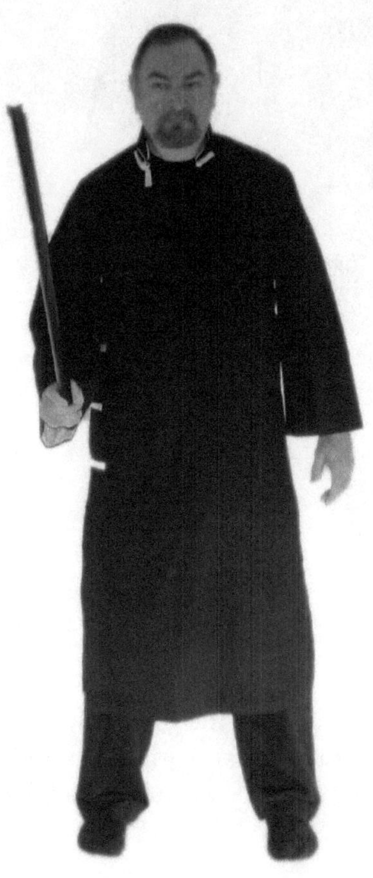

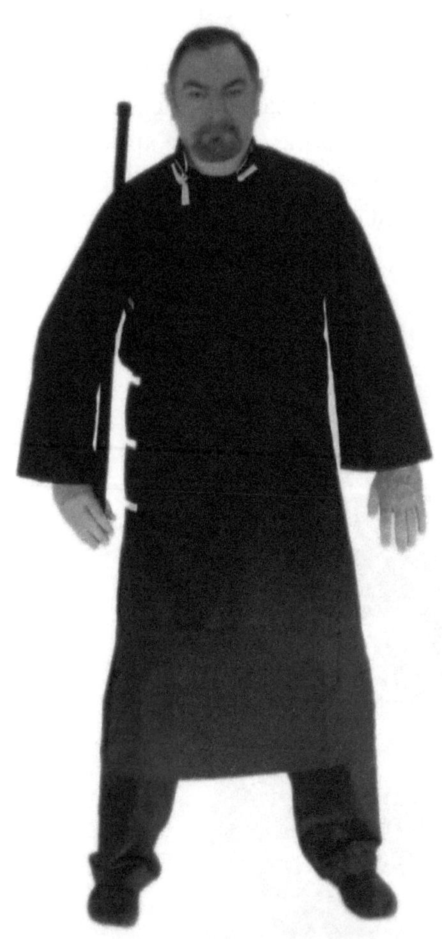

Strike Upward and Kick with Left Foot - West

The cane drops with the release of the wrist down to the right foot. The cane then circles upward using an underhand grip to a standing position to the southwest and the left foot follows with a low left-foot kick looking like a raised foot.

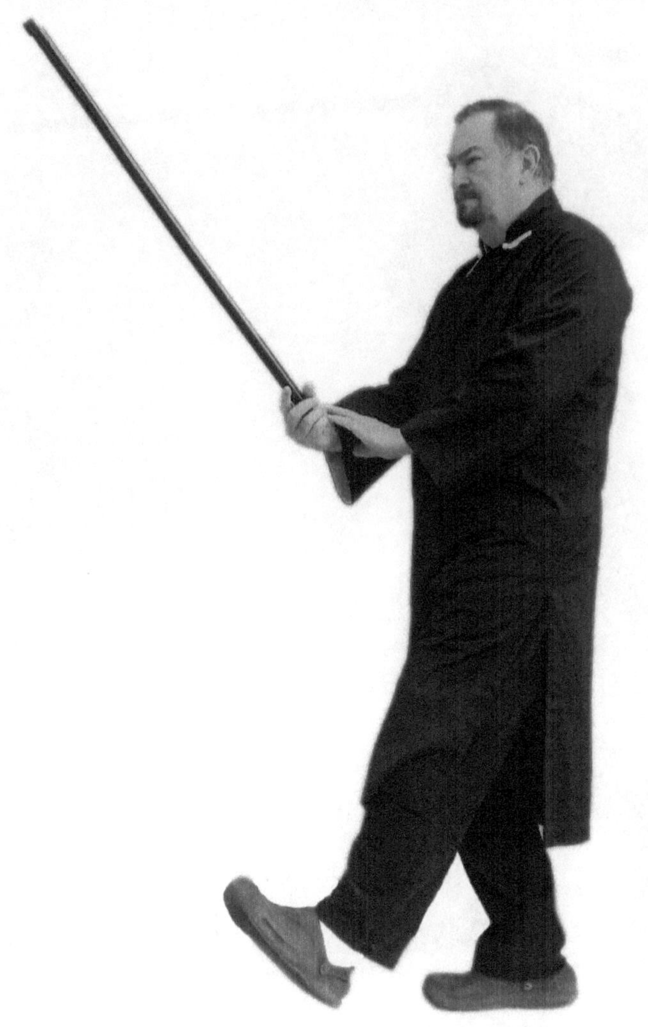

Strike Horizontally

The left foot steps pointing to the Southwest. The right foot steps to the Northwest and weight shifts to the left leg. The cane turns and strikes to the Northwest striking with the cane level at head height and the left hand over the right wrist for support.

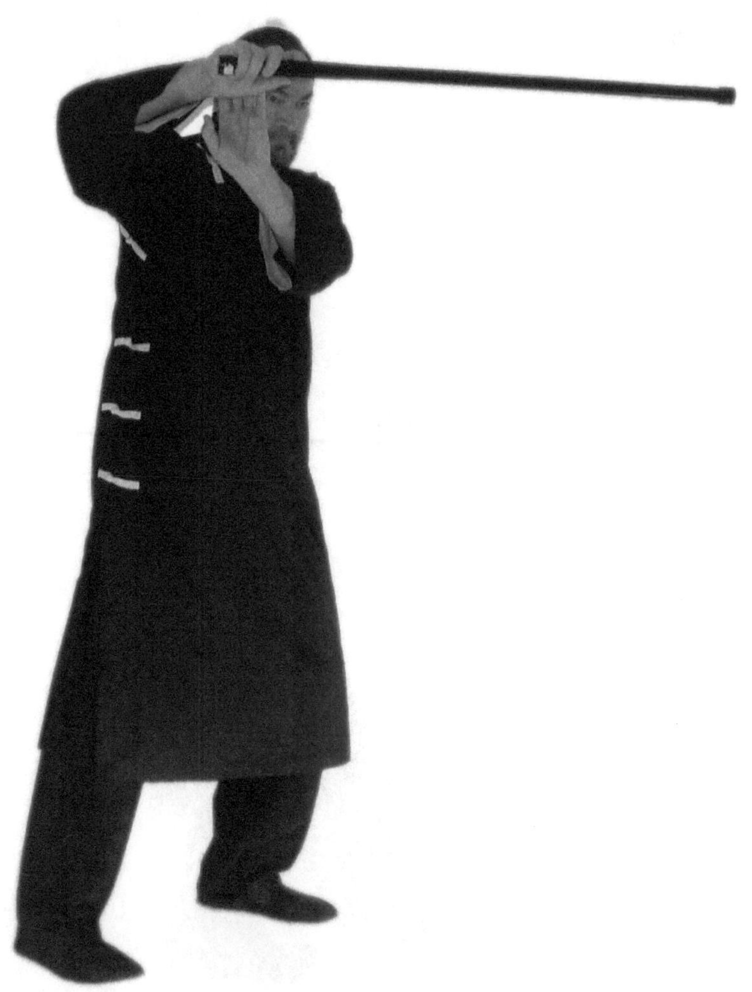

The upper body comes back to face the west and the left hand slides out to the other end of the cane. The left leg steps back as body retreats backward with the shift of the weight to the right foot. The left foot steps forward and the weight shifts back to the left foot and then strikes / blocks to the west with a two-handed cane held level at shoulder height.

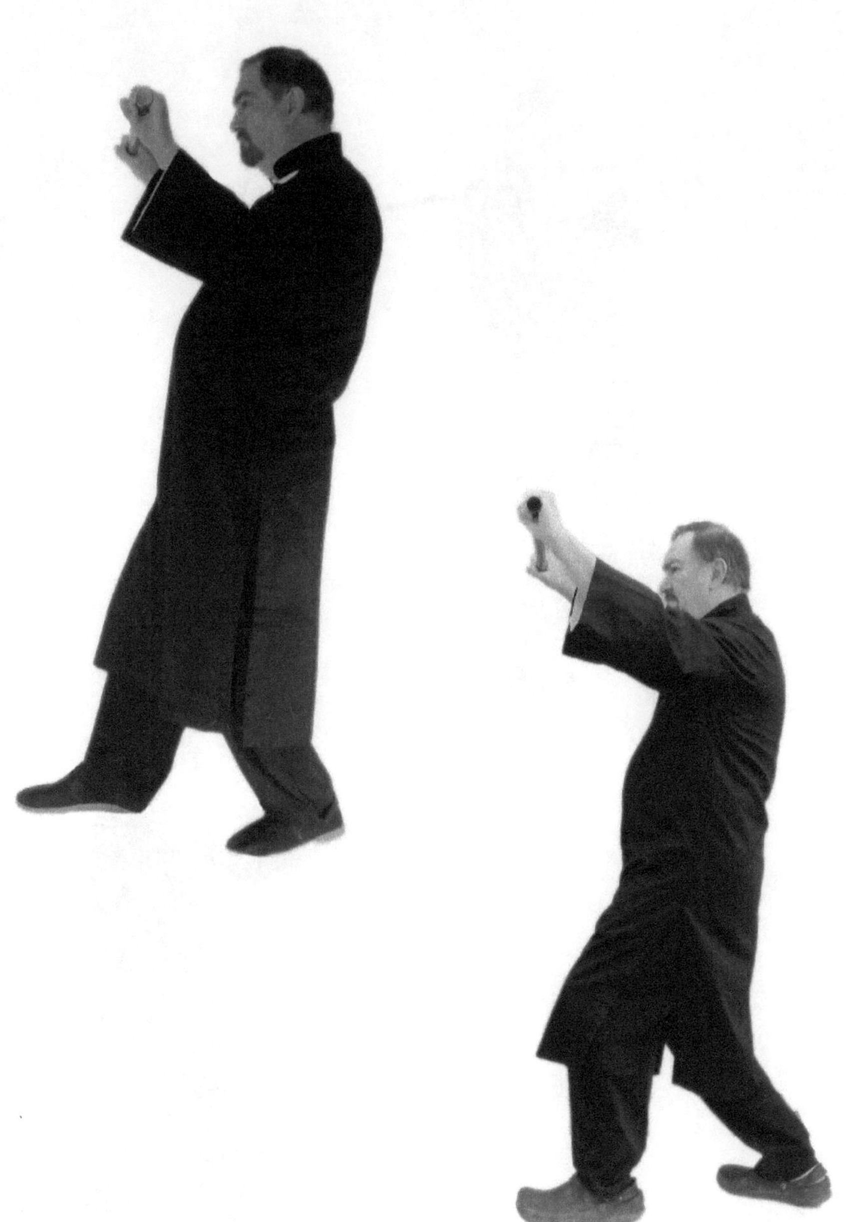

The left hand leaves the cane and the right hand circles the cane inside and to the back as the left foot moves back in a retreating action. The cane comes back on the right side as the left foot steps forward. The left hand opens and strikes with the palm as the cane strikes to the west at the opponent's ears.

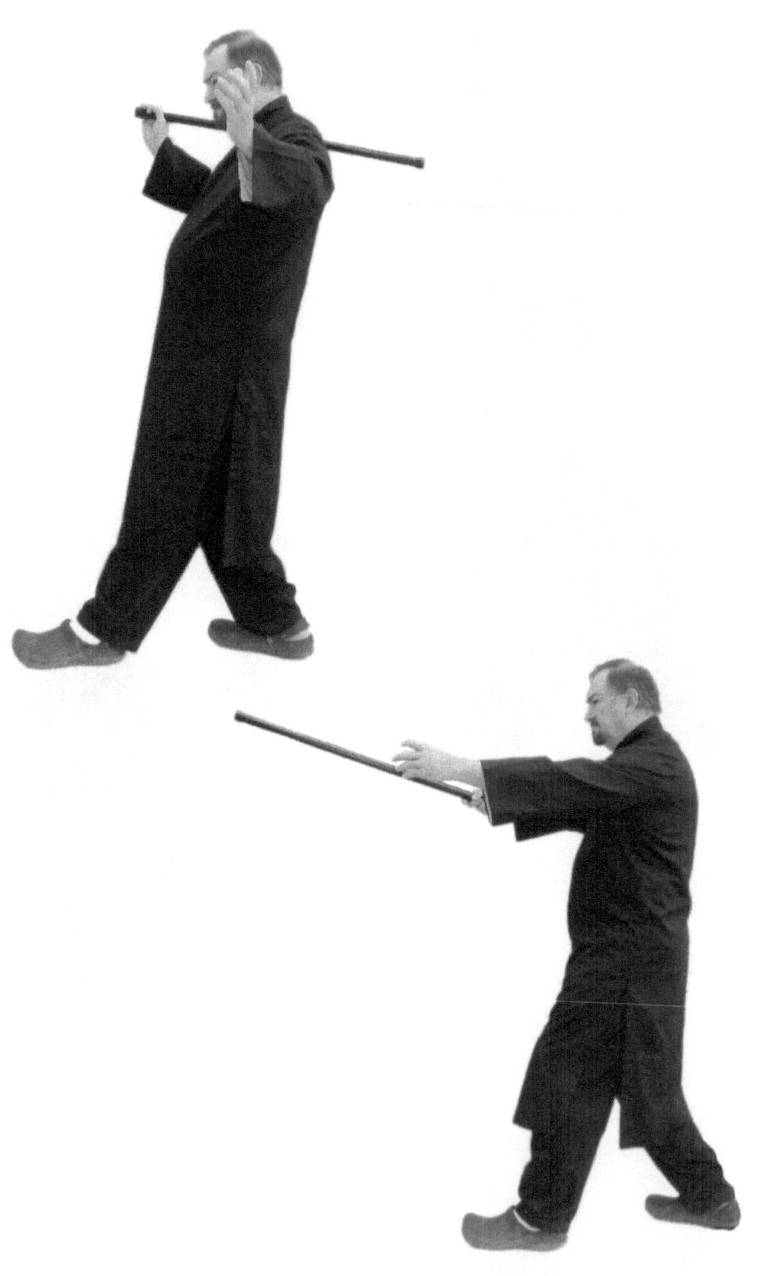

Hook Hand Step and strike with Cane downward – West

The left foot steps forward and the left hand reaches out with a hook hand[5] on the inside of the opponent's body. The right hand circles the cane downward. The cane strikes over the top with a downward action to the West as the left hand comes to the back of the player outstretched to the East.

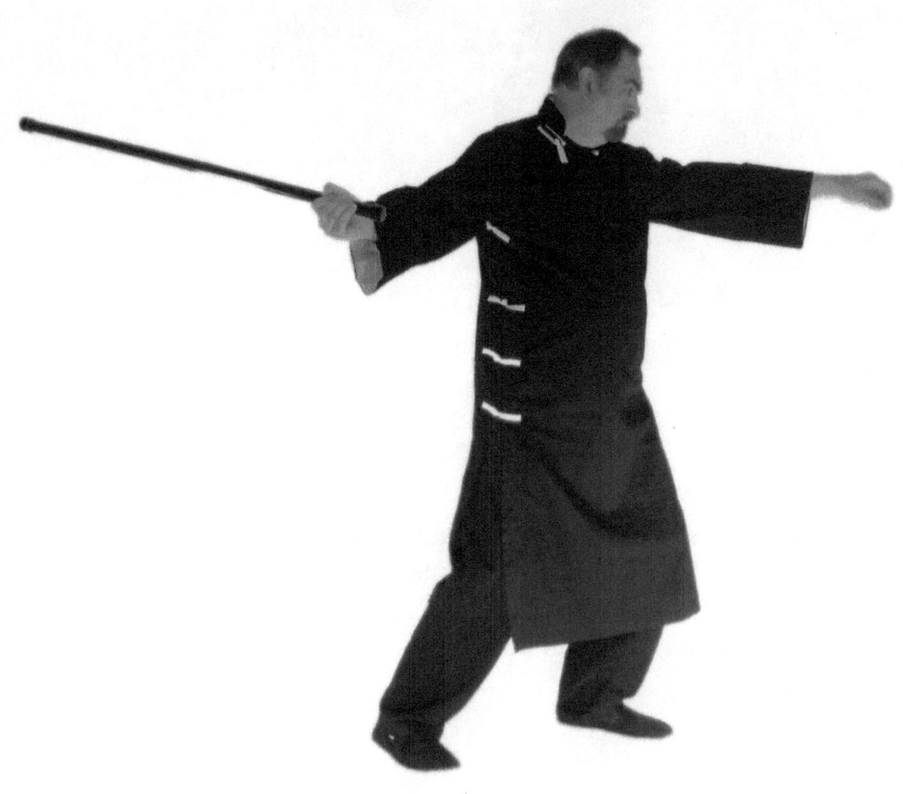

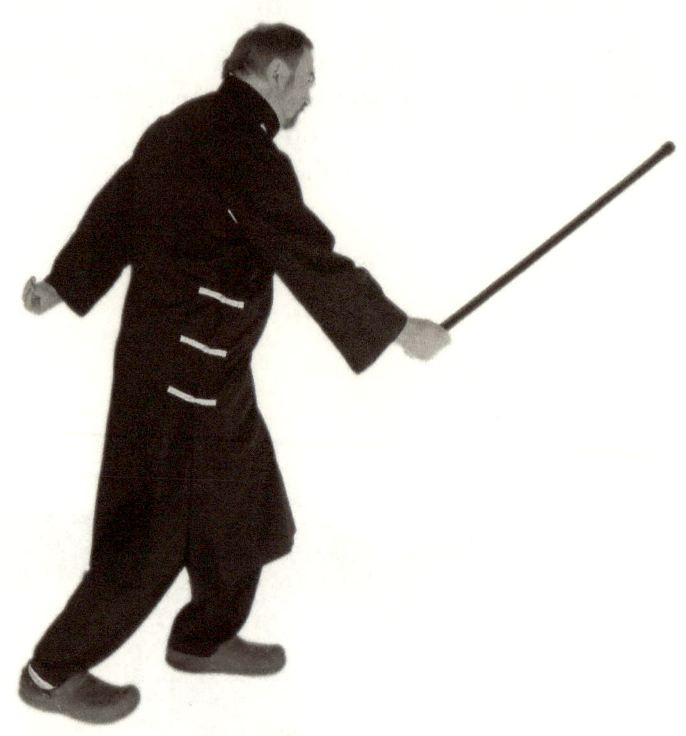

Cover and Underhand strike - West

Swing the cane out and over the left shoulder in circle covering the back shifting the weight on the left leg. Short step with the right foot pointed north and sit down on left leg. Cane swings underhand to the west with the left hand stretched to the right hand palm down.

Left Cover

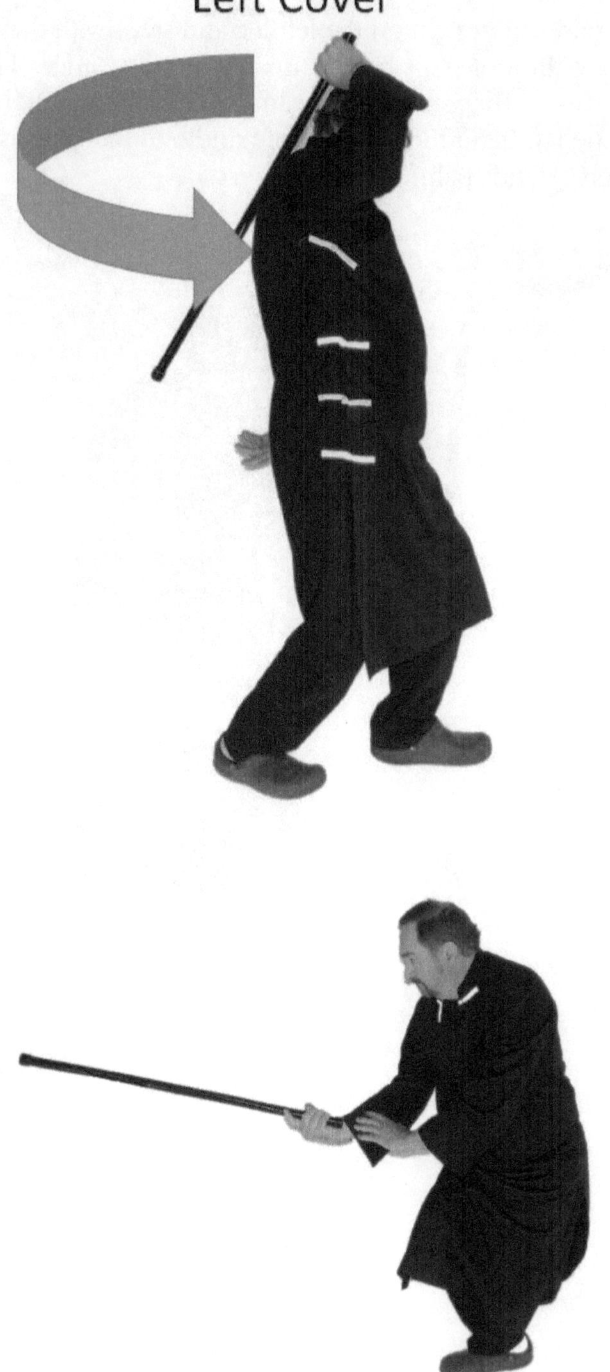

The player raises up weight on the left leg and steps with the right foot pointing north. The right foot steps behind in a cross step stance. The player strikes down to the west as they sit into a squatting stance the weight remaining of on the left leg. The left hand moves into the handle of the cane as it swings by the waist and then extends palm up to the West

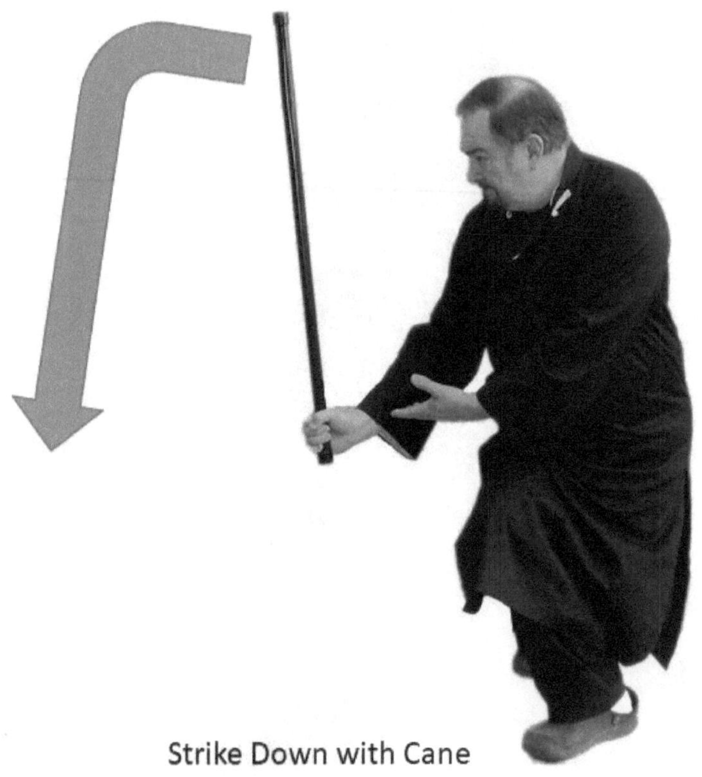

Strike Down with Cane

Section 2

Strike upwards and kick with the Right foot - Northeast

The player swings the cane downward and up with a standing cane to the Northeast corner as they pivot on the left foot and raise the right in a kick to the East. The left hand goes to the right wrist. The right foot kicks with the heel slightly raised. (Mirror image of section 1 movement)[6]

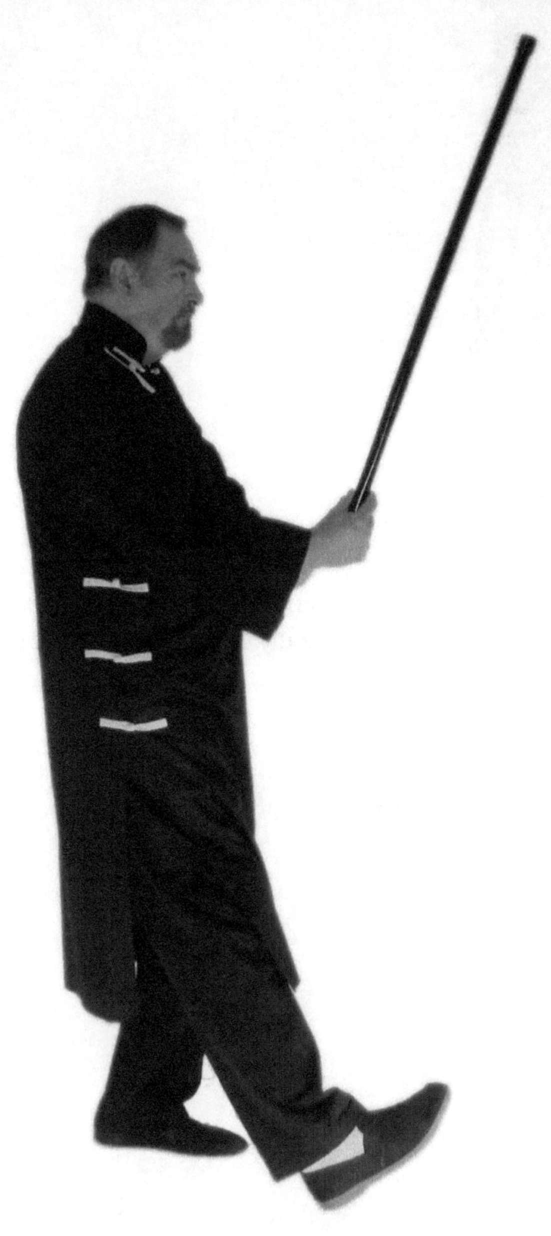

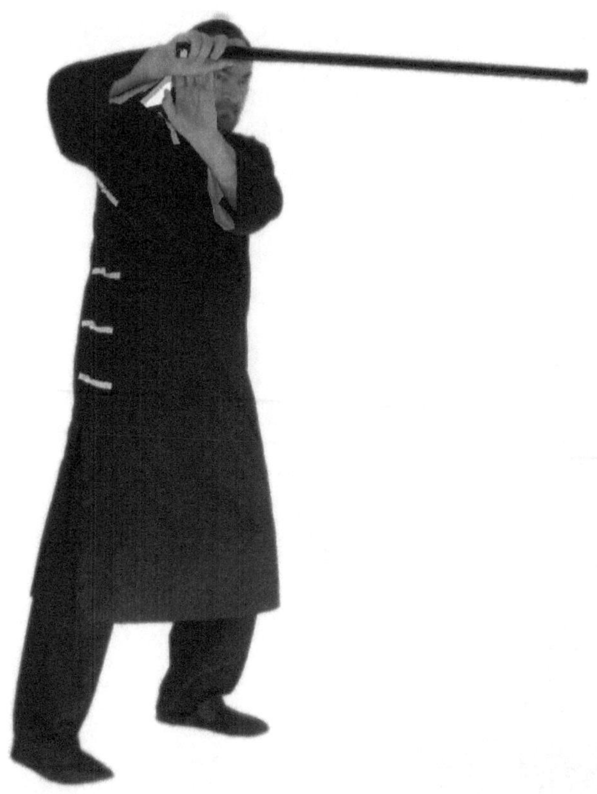

The player steps with the right foot pointing to the Southeast and shifts the weight to that leg. The cane strikes horizontally to the Southeast at shoulder height.

Retreat and block with two Hands – East

The upper body comes back to face the east and the left hand slides out to the other end of the cane. The body retreats backward with the shift of the weight and then strikes/blocks to the west with a two-handed cane held level and the right foot forward. (Mirror image of section 1 movement)

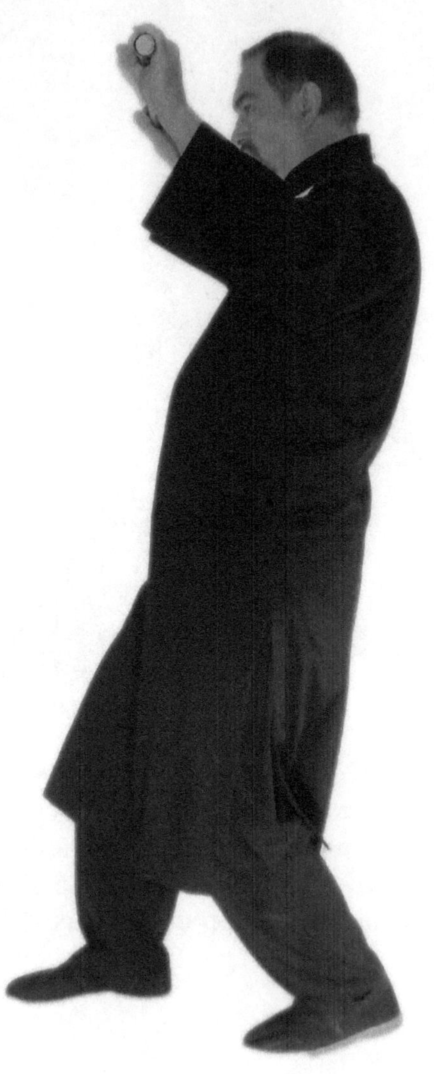

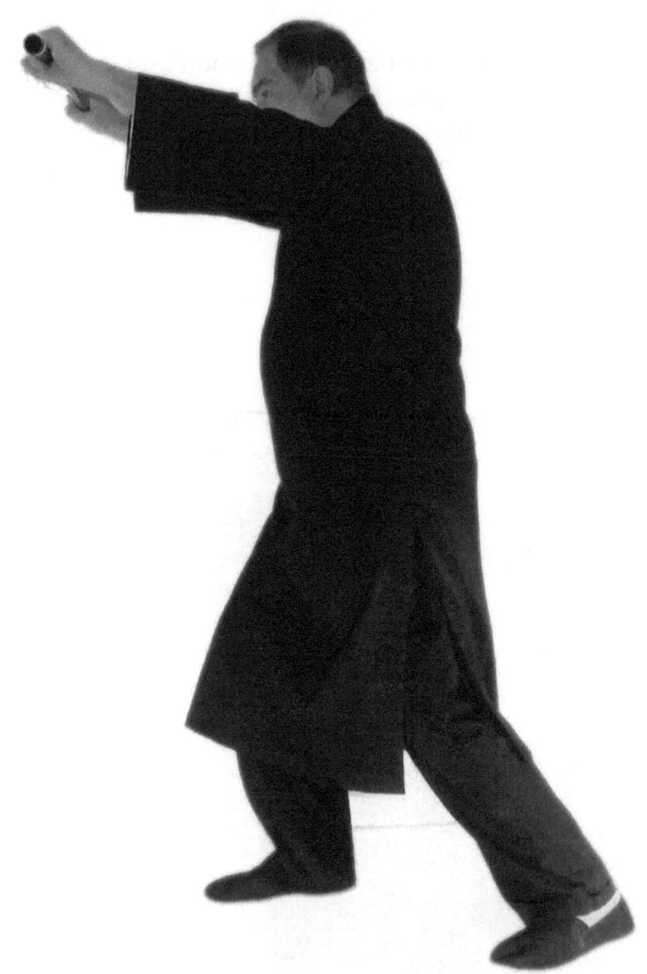

The left hand lets the cane go and the right hand circles the cane inside and to the back as the right foot steps back. The cane comes back on the right side as the right foot steps forward. The left hand opens and strikes with the palm as the cane strikes to the east at the opponent's ears. (Mirror image of section 1 movement)

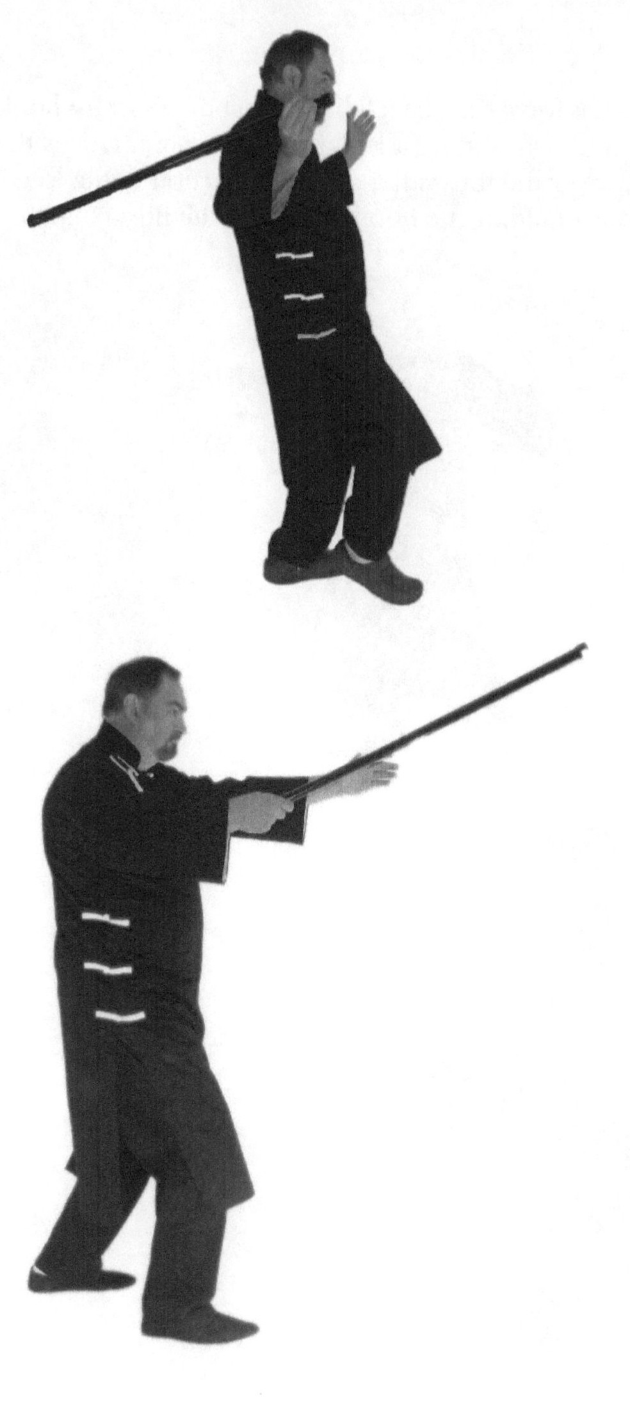

Hook Hand, Step and strikes with Cane downward – East

The left foot steps forward. The left hand reaches out with a hook hand. The player steps forward with the right leg as the right hand circles the cane downward and strikes over the top with a downward action to the West. The left hand goes to the west holding the hook hand with the fingers up.

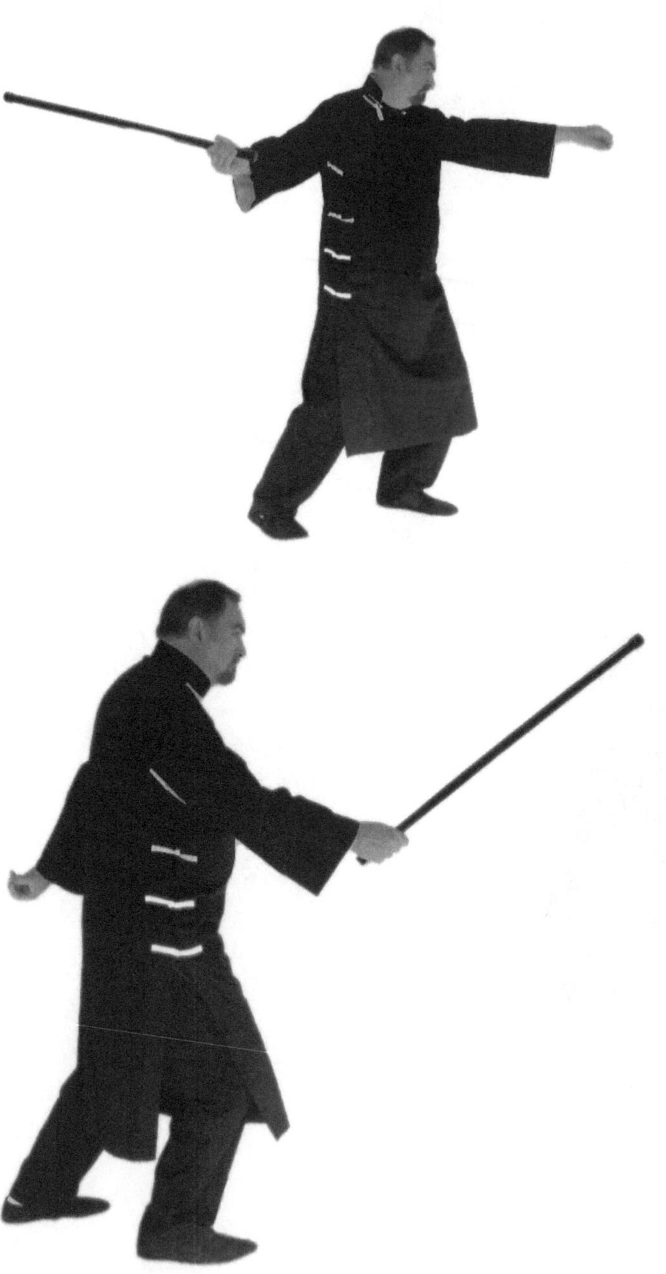

Cover and Underhand Strike

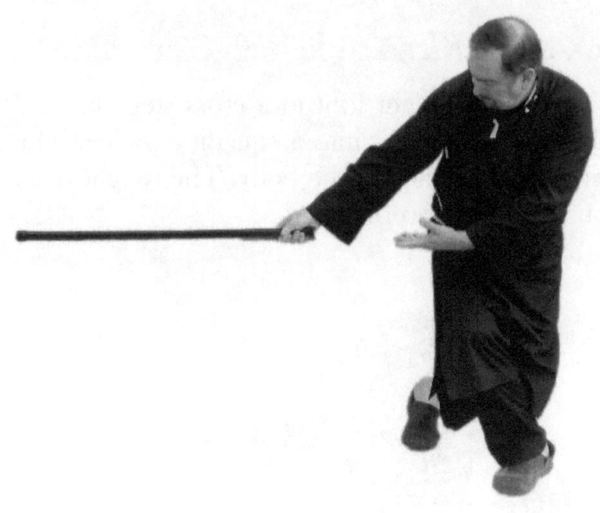

Right Cover

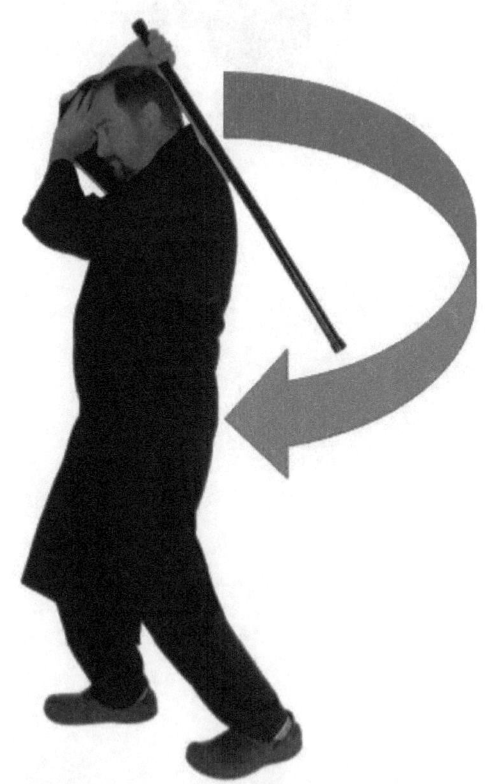

The cane circles over the right shoulder as the weight shifts back on the left leg. The right leg steps back and then forward pointing North. The left foot steps behind the right as the cane strikes out underhand to the East. The left hand assumes a palm up posture.

Step behind, sit and underhand strike with Cane - East

The left foot steps behind the right foot in a cross step stance. The player strikes upward to the East as they sit into a squatting stance. The left hand, palm up creates a circular shape across the body. The weight is on the right foot. (Mirror image of section 1 movement)

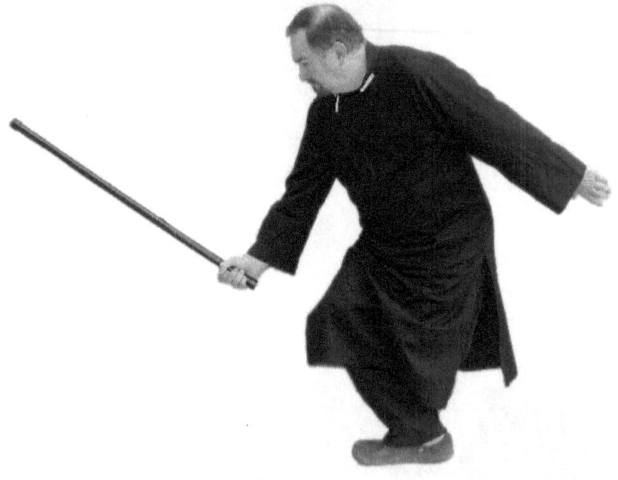

Section 3

Stand the cane – East

Shift the weight to the left leg. Step to the side with the right foot to a low horse stance. The right wrist snaps the cane into a vertical position. The left hand covers the right wrist.

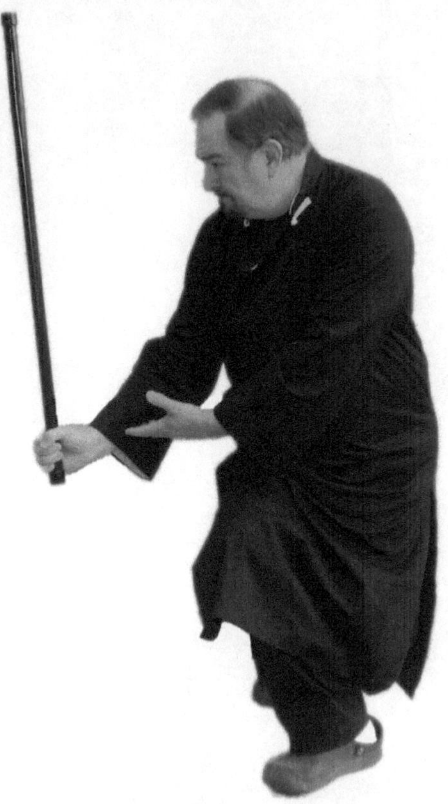

The player stands to a medium horse stance. The left hand grasps bottom of the cane. Both hands hold the cane like a baseball bat.

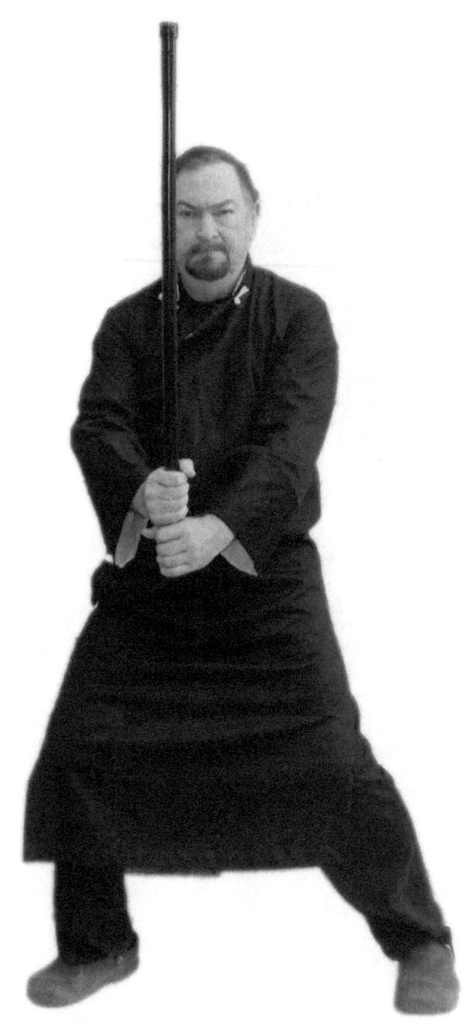

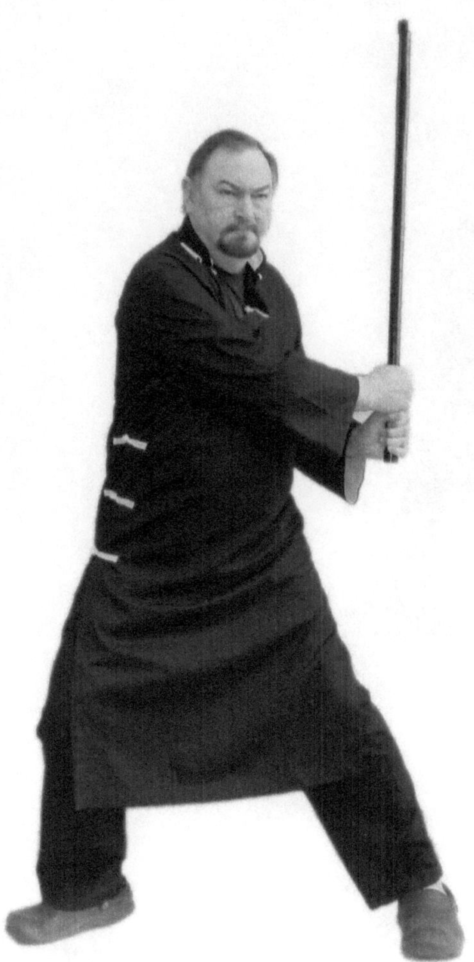

Standing cane strikes Right

The player shifts the weight to the left with the waist turning to the left and the cane remaining upright and strikes to the southeast with the vertical cane as the right foot slides besides the left foot.

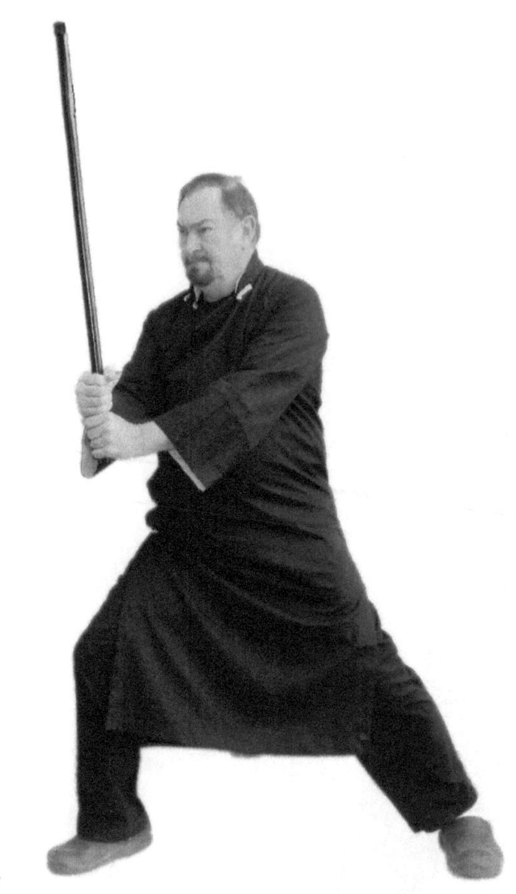

Step to the Left

Step with the right foot to the North

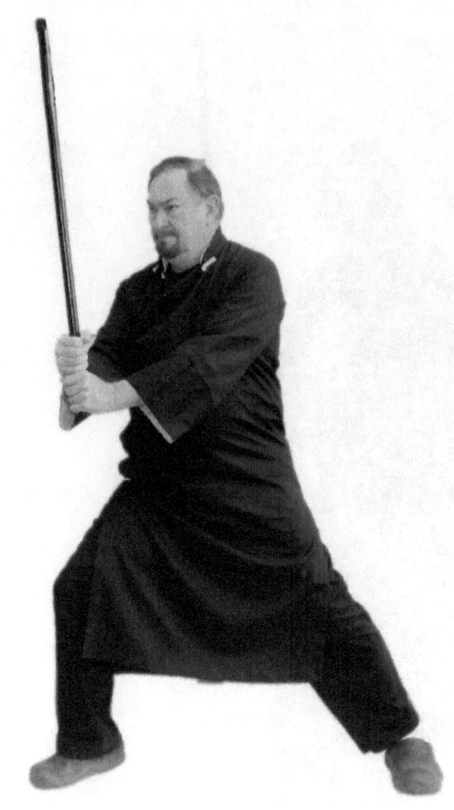

Standing cane Strikes Left

Shift the weight to the right foot with the waist turning to the North West striking with a vertical cane.

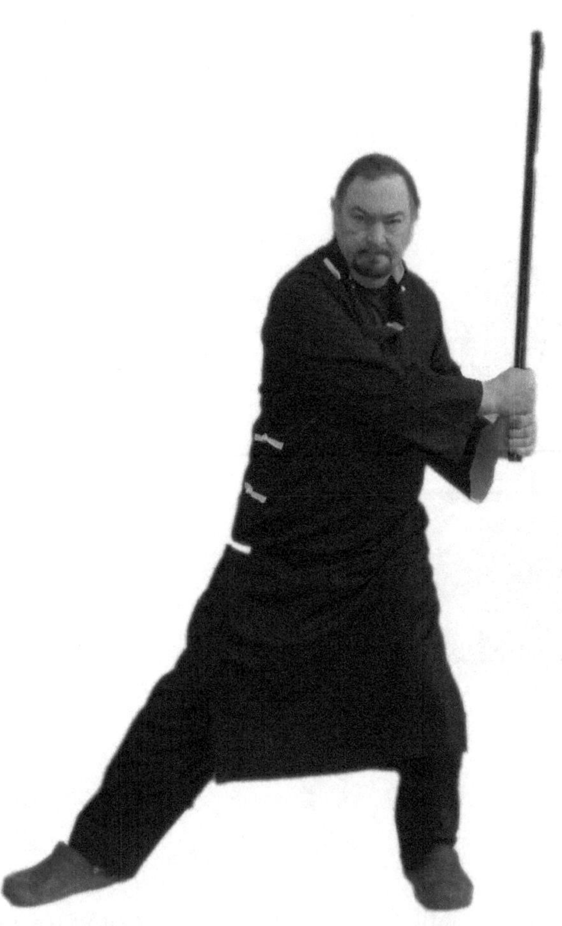

Step to the Left

Cover and Underhand strike

The cane circles over the back, drops down, and swings underhand to the Southwest as the left leg steps out to the Southwest and the cane strikes upward.

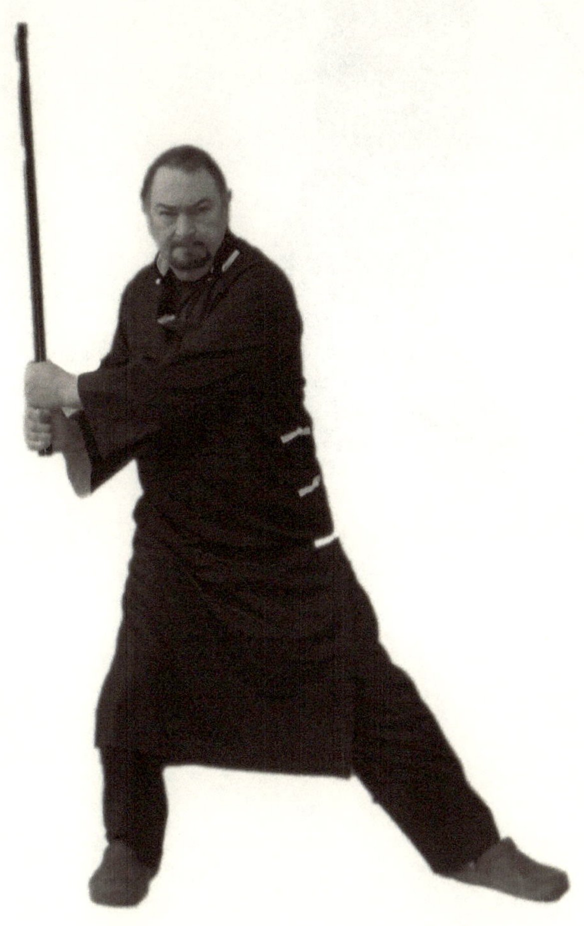

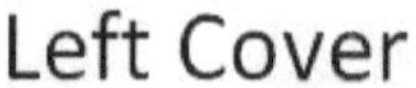

Left Cover

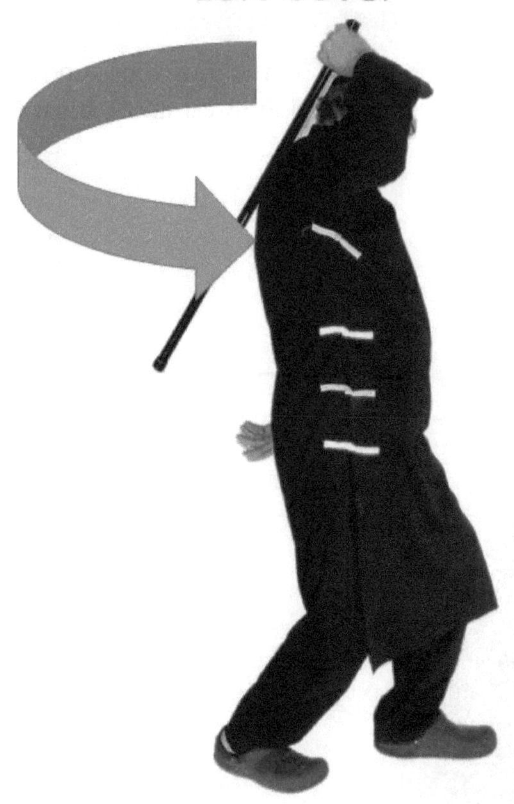

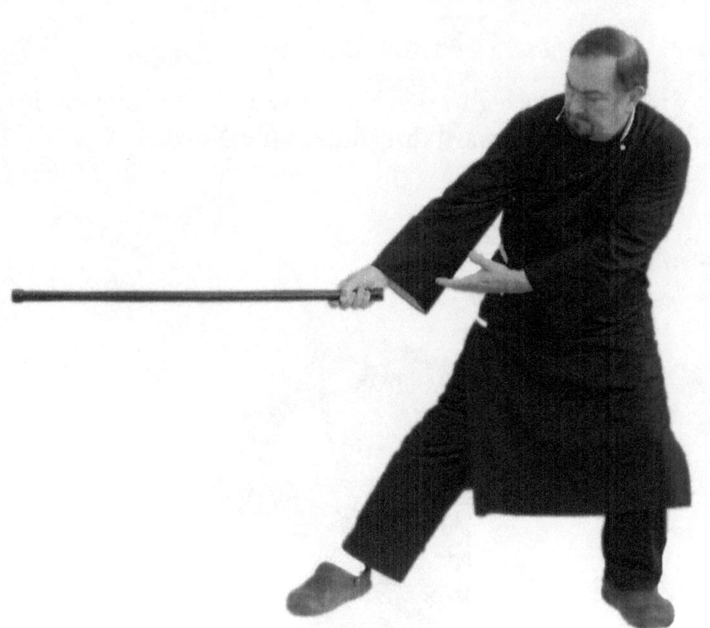

Step to the Right

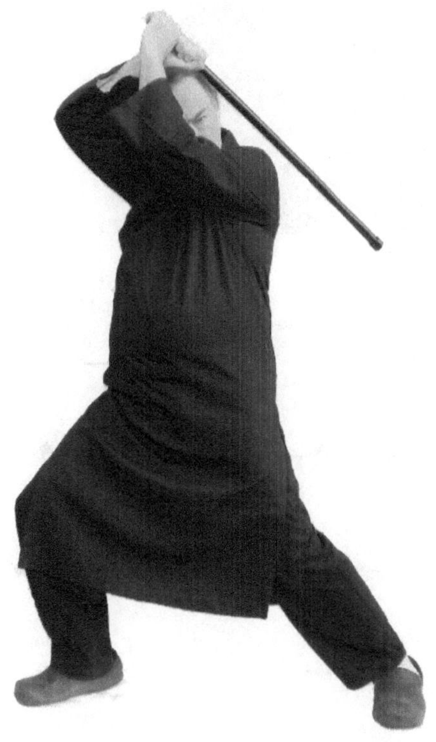

Step out with the right leg to the Northeast and the cane circles over the back and strikes out in an upward direction to the Northeast.

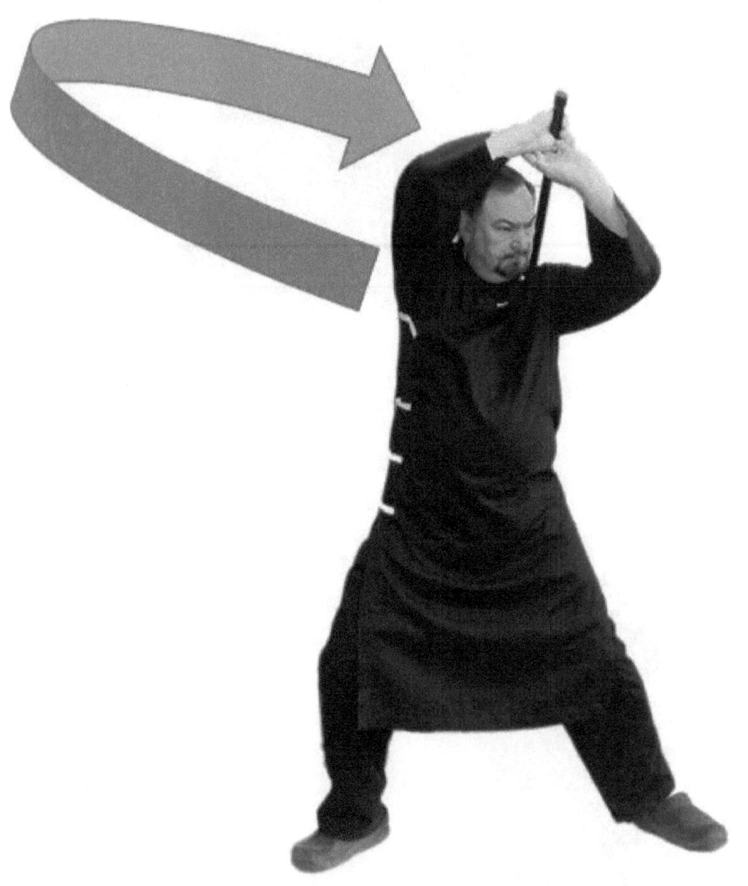

Circling the back 2

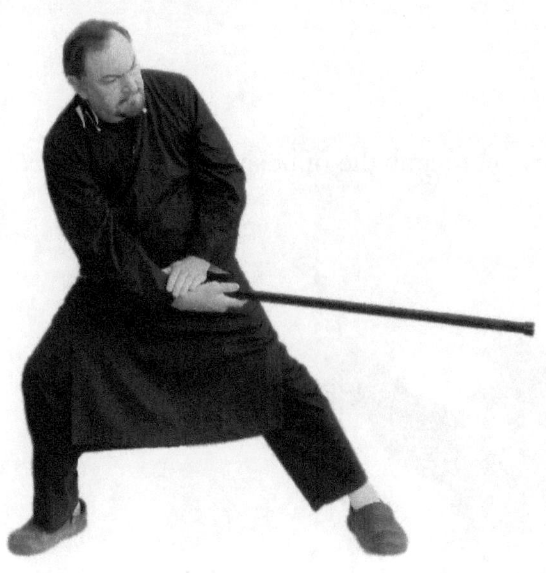

Overhand Strike left hand behind back – Northwest

Step with the left foot. Step behind the left leg with the right as the player squats. The cane circles up and strikes down to the west as the player squats down with the left hand coming in to support the player's right wrist.

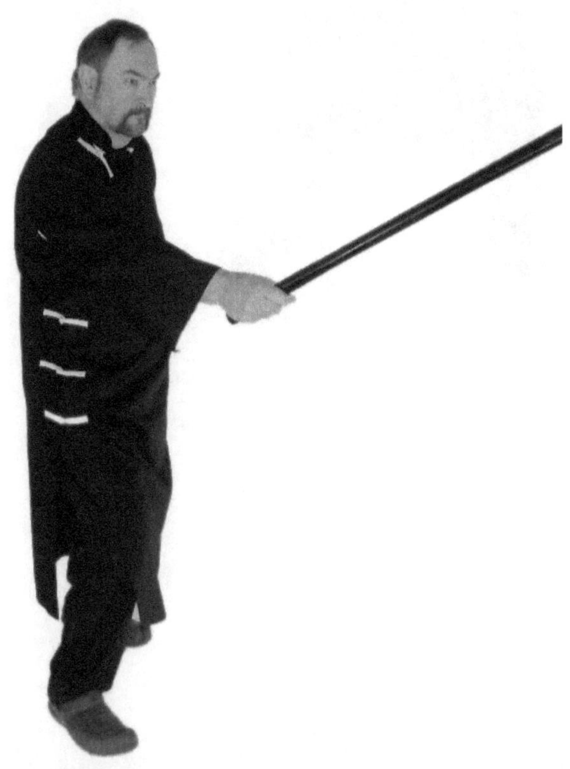

The left hand slides out to grab the opposite end of the cane.

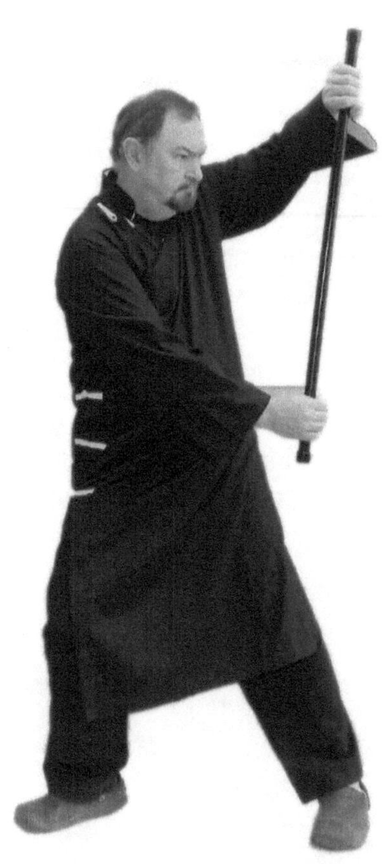

Fold cane under the arm – North

The left hand continues bringing the end of the cane in and up under the arm to the armpit and the left hand then goes to the left side at the waist.

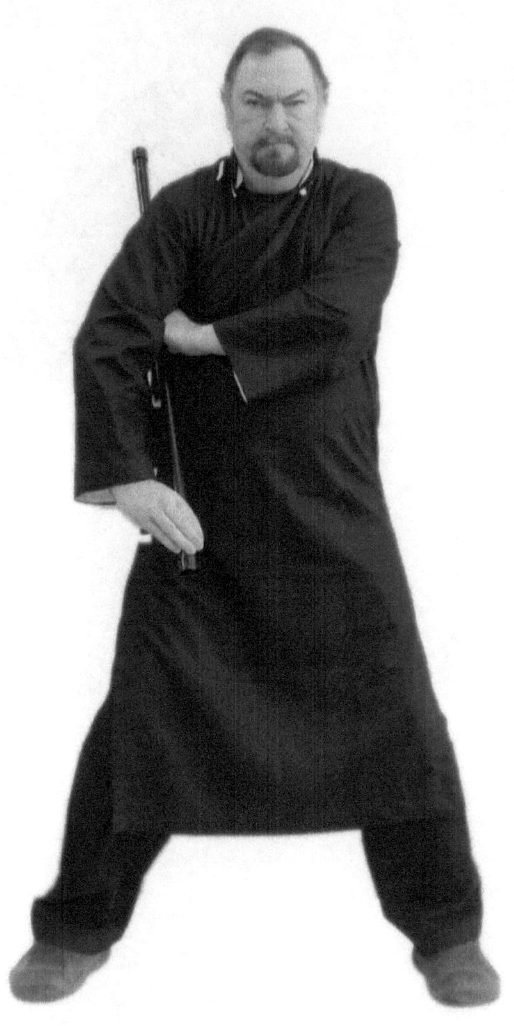

The cane swings down and out to the north to waist level continues making an outside circle going up and back to the side and comes down to rest at the outside of the right foot.

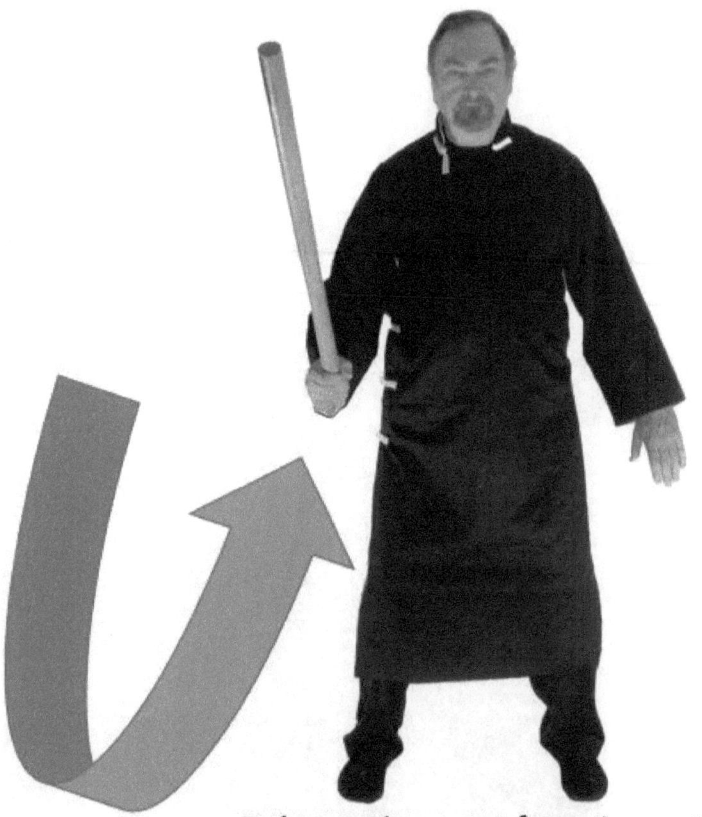

Release the cane from in nest

The cane finishes its circle to the foot. This ends the form in its starting position. In a formal presentation, the player would bow to the audience.

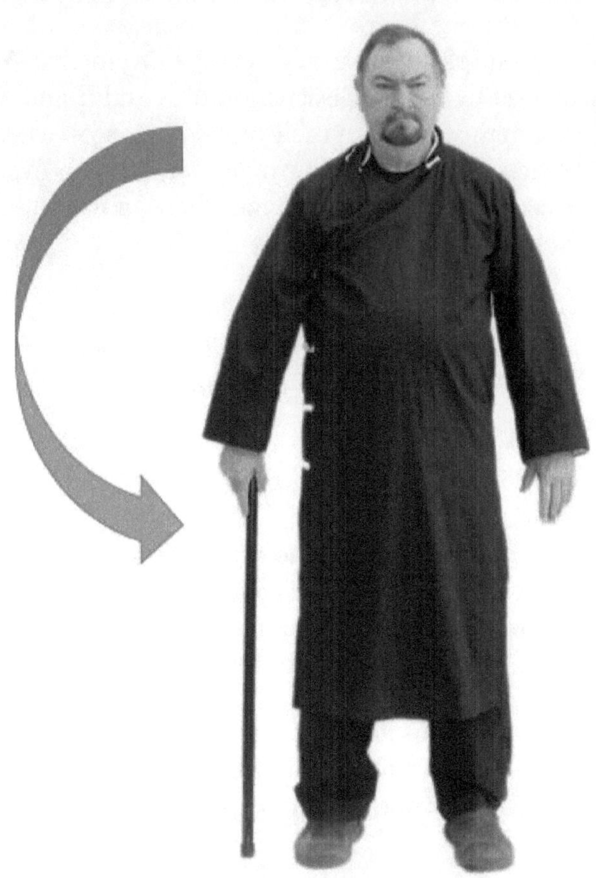

Cane comes to rest

Two person sets

There are many sets where two people can practice in real time to use the cane. Safety is the most important concern since a strike from a cane can cause injury. Use protective equipment and soft canes. The PVC pipe is a good alternative but still can hurt. Go slow and wear head and mouth protection.

There is one example of a simple set of movements. Any of these techniques can make a set by using a designation of A and B and wait until the other player has had a chance to finish their movement. Stop when needed to discuss options with each movement. How many ways can an overhand strike be used? Find them all, practice each, and then move to add another movement. Slow, internal and fun!

As a preview of the advanced volume, think of where are movements that relate to other weapons – they are there. Remember techniques from Sword or knife practice. Play with it with the canes since many can be quite valuable techniques in the cane form.

A Two-person set

A starts from the ready position and raises the cane up to a horizontal position at chest level with the end of the cane pointing at B. As the cane is raised, the left hand moves in and the palm of the left hand reinforces the end of the cane. A then pushes the cane forward towards B's chest in an attack.

B raises the cane up to a standing position as the left hand goes to hold the bottom of the cane. B then turns their waist to the left swinging the cane vertically across in front of their body to intercept the strike and direct the cane away.

A moves the cane in the direction to B's strike using the momentum of the strike to swing the cane out and down and strike at B's knee.

B raises their leg to avoid the strike and swings their cane to their right and downward and meets A's swing. Both canes are cross in a downward direction.

B steps down with their raised leg and raises the cane straight up to strike at A's torso.

A steps back and brings their cane up to strike B's cane from below.

Both A and B step back to a basic standing position with each cane circling up and down the outside of their body to end at the starting position.

The End

It never ends it just takes another breath

The various movements of the cane are covered in this volume. These details only cover the basic movements. The path to knowledge starts with the initial steps and movements. Play with the ideas and sets in this volume. The movements do not have to be perfect just grab the end of a stick and remember the rules of Tai Chi Chuan – slow and mind intent. Practice techniques in this volume and develop routines for practice. The second volume in the Cane

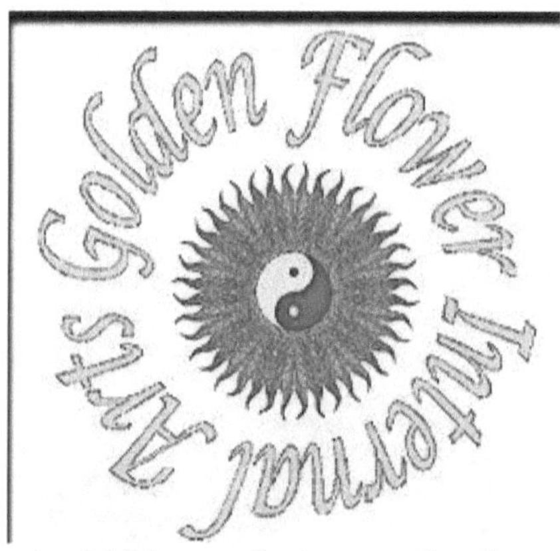

Series discusses the hidden techniques of strikes, locks, and throws. Look for more volumes in the Internal Arts series.

The Author

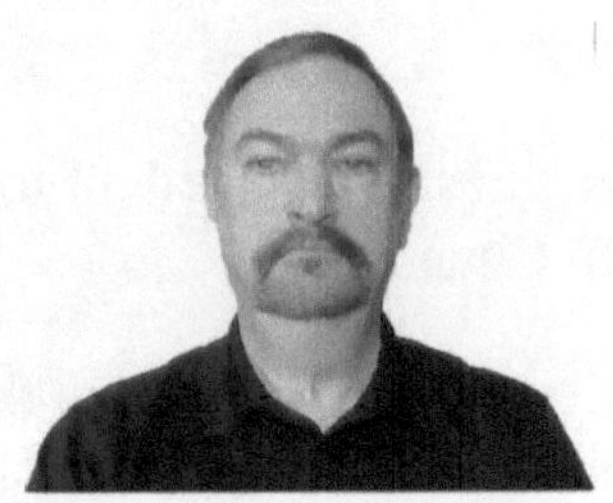

Robert George Downey (Sifu Bob) studied meditation and the martial arts most of his life. He has been a dedicated student of meditation and Internal Arts since 1970. His study started with a wide variety of systems and then focused on the Internal Arts. Sifu Bob has developed an understanding of their associated practices – meditation, qigong, and Traditional Chinese medicine - that leads to increased skills in the arts and improved health. He has studied extensively with Grandmasters Chen and Liang. He studied and practiced Taoist Arts, Tibetan Buddhism, and Zen Meditation. He has been teaching martial arts, meditation, and qigong since the 1980s and is a co-founder of South Shore Internal Arts Association, a martial arts school that has presented seminars in the Internal Arts since the 1970s. Sifu Bob currently runs Golden Flower Internal Arts and teaches private lessons. His practice includes Tai Chi Chuan and Bagua, meditation and qigong practice, teaching and writing every day.

Goldenflowerinternalarts

Mail

Goldenflowerinternalarts

Mail

End Notes

---

[1] Cane as a teaching tool – a cane is excellent to show posture and knee alignment in teaching Tai Chi Chuan.

[2] Waist The waist in the oriental martial arts is at the hip level and not at the stomach level. Bending at the stomach level may injure the lower back

[3] Tai Chi Volumes – Two volumes on the art of Tai Chi Chuan are scheduled to be published by Golden Flower Internal Arts and may be available by the time you are reading this note. See the web site or check on Amazon.

[4] Safety Equipment – Whenever practicing with a partner the use of safety equipment is essential. A mouthpiece at a minimum and headgear and elbow pads are great additions to cane fencing practice.

[5] Hook Hand – the hook hand is often in the Martial Arts. The fingers all gather and touch at the tips and drop down. The wrist is straight to prevent damage and to add to strength.

[6] Yes, two sides, this cane form has two sides to the form. North is the starting position and then the form moves to the West. It then turns and moves to the East. Between these directional movements are transitional movements. As you practice the form, you will see the first section repeated in section 2 with changes to the feet. Try each movement doing the left side and then the right side one after the other. This will aid in the learning process. Do not be concerned if you do a left or right sided posture on the wrong side. Just continue and have fun.

9 781795 851602